All Sickness is Home Sickness

Also by Dianne M. Connelly

Traditional Acupuncture: The Law of the Five Elements

All Sickness is Home Sickness

dianne m. connelly

Artwork by John Levering

ISBN 0-912379-02-2

Grateful acknowledgment is made for permission to reprint excerpts from the following works:

Overnight in the Guest House of the Mystic by Dick Allen. Published by the Louisiana State University Press, 1984. Reprinted by permission of the publisher.

"from spiralling ecstatically this" copyright © 1956 by E. E. Cummings. Reprinted from his volume *Complete Poems 1913-1962* by permission of Harcourt Brace Jovanovich, Inc.

"home means that" copyright © 1958 by E. E. Cummings.Reprinted from his volume *Complete Poems 1913-1962* by permission of Harcourt Brace Jovanovich, Inc.

"love is a place" reprinted from *No Thanks* by E. E. Cummings by permission of Liveright Publishing Corporation. Copyright 1935 by E. E. Cummings. Copyright © 1968 by Marion Morehouse Cummings. Copyright © 1973, 1978 by the Trustees for the E. E. Cummings Trust. Copyright © 1973, 1978 by George James Firmage.

Easy Death by Da Free John. Copyright 1983 by the Johannine Daist Communion. Published by the Dawn Horse Press. Reprinted by permission of the publisher.

"Ash Wednesday" in *Collected Poems 1909-1962* by T. S. Eliot, copyright 1936 by Harcourt Brace Jovanovich, Inc.; copyright © 1963, 1964 by T. S. Eliot. Reprinted by permission of the publisher.

Four Quartets by T. S. Eliot, copyright 1943 by T. S. Eliot, renewed 1971 by Esme Valerie Eliot. Reprinted by permission of Harcourt Brace Jovanovich, Inc.

"The Death of the Hired Man" in *The Poetry of Robert Frost*, edited by Edward Connery Lathem. Copyright 1930, 1939, © 1969 by Holt, Rinehart and Winston. Copyright © 1958 by Robert Frost. Copyright © 1967 by Leslie Frost Ballantine. Reprinted by permission of Henry Holt and Company.

"Footnote to Howl" from *Collected Poems 1947-1980* by Allen Ginsberg. Copyright © 1955 by Allen Ginsberg. Reprinted by permission of Harper and Row Publishers, Inc.

(continued on page 166)

Dedication

Mick - Michael W. Kilchenstein, M.D.

Your love calls me home. I am listening.

Acknowledgments

To acknowledge is to admit to be true. I admit to be true that life is given to me by others. And so, to my fellow travelers with whom I am home enroute, I give thanks to you for my life:

- Irene, for being my mother.
- Blaize, Jade, and Caeli, for being my children.
- Andy, Jack, Jerry, Steve, Peg, for being my brothers and sister.
- Bob, for being my partner.
- Mary Ellen, for being my "midwife" for this book.
- John, for being my artist.
- Guy, for being my copy editor.
- Flor, for being my benefactress.
- Barbara, Betsy, Bob, Carol, Colin, Debbie, Diane, Don, Elaine, Fernando, Frank, Freida, Fritz, Harwood, Jan, Jane, Janet, Jed, Jenny, Jim, Joan, John, Judy, Karen, Pere Larre, Larry, Lee, Lillian, Linda Joy, Lorraine, Lynn, Mark, Martha, Mary, Matthew, Meriel, Nikki, Pat, Paula, Rachel, Rollo, Sherman, Stephanie, Stephen, Susan, Tiffany, Vickie, Werner, JRW, Yola, for being my friends, fellow board members and mentors.

- The faculty of the Traditional Acupuncture Institute — Beverly, Bill, Bob, Charlotte, Cyrie, Erica, Gary, Haig, Jack, Jane, Jim, Jon, Julia, Khosrow, Leslie, Marion, Melissa, Sarah, Zoe—for being my colleagues.
- The student body of the Traditional Acupuncture Institute, for teaching me.
- The staff of the Centre for Traditional Acupuncture, for taking care of me.
- My patients, for trusting me.
- The thousands of people all over the world who have my first book, *Traditional Acupuncture: The Law of the Five Elements*, for reading me.

To all of you—without your listening, I cannot speak. Thank you for my life.

Contents

A Note From
Dianne M. Connelly

I am home, I am home, I am home . . .

— Florida Scott-Maxwell

The lives of the saints were important to me as a child. I read and reread the life stories of these most amazing human beings, people who would do things beyond the ordinary, people whose lives had enormous influence on others. I was in awe. I read, not knowing that I was looking for something.

One day I discovered some words from the Confessions of St. Augustine, lamentations from a man whose profligate life had disguised his powerful love:

> Late have I loved Thee,
> O Beauty so Ancient and so New
> Late have I loved Thee.
> . . . .
> Our hearts were made for Thee, O Lord,
> and they are restless until they rest in Thee.

Augustine awakened to something beyond what he had previously seen. He recognized something crucial for living his life. He had been living with a "missing." His whole life was a desideratum. His thirst was quenchable by nothing that he already knew. His actions had been directed by his limited vision of life's possibilities. He had used pain and pleasure as guides from experience to experience, never quite satisfied in his desires. What he discovered was something else, some "I know not what" beyond where he already "lived."

To me, a young reader of this great saint's life, I could see that he was unaware of what he did not know up until a moment of vision that altered his entire life. It was easier for me to see how a man as great as Augustine could express his love into life than it was to see how I, a little girl, reading this great man, could express my love into life. He used the language of God, of Lord, of beauty in his awakening to creation. He spoke of his coming home to the Love of his life, to the Beauty without which he was forever restless. His words of proclamation and lament spoke for me too: "Late have I loved Thee."

In his words were a declaration of arrival. In his arriving, I opened to my own homecoming, a collective human homecoming. If all sickness is homesickness, then all healing is coming home, and like Augustine, I can bring forth into life whatever has been missing, I can call into being an opening for which there are no words, I can begin to dwell in the poetry of existence.

This conversation is an ongoing dialogue, having begun long ago for me and continuing with the Jesuits in my college years. One of those years I spent living and studying in Rome, engaging in what were deeply inspiring discourses on being and being in the world.

The work of two men in particular inspired me past old patterns of thought. One was a man who lived in Italy during the time I was there. His name was Bernard Lonergan, a Jesuit, who wrote a book called *Insight: A Study of Human Understanding*. The other was a man, also of the Society of Jesus, whose name was Pierre Teilhard de Chardin. Although I did not personally know Teilhard, he became my mentor.

His thoughts were acts of creation, questions into the nature of life, of matter, of God, of man. His inquiry was not a search for answers, but rather an invitation to investigate issues at the heart of being a human being, grounded in matter.

Teilhard spoke: "I live at the heart of a single unique element at the centre of the universe and present in each part of it: personal Love and cosmic Power." He continues: "God, who is eternal Being-in-it-self, is, one might say, everywhere in process of formation *for us*."

I saw through the eyes of this human being what life might be like as a creative act, as a continual and evolving creation of our holiness, our wholeness—life as a hymn to the universe. His *Mass on the World* proclaims: "We are all of us together carried in the one world-womb; yet each of us is our own little microcosm in which the Incarnation is wrought independently with degrees of intensity, and shades that are incommunicable . . . . I have been brought to the point where I can no longer see anything, nor any longer breathe, outside that 'milieu' in which all is made one . . . . radiant bliss: to have found the Word and so be able to achieve the mastery of matter . . . ."

Throughout my entire life I have only ever wanted to love and to live from that love. It is love which is my constancy in a day—like a golden thread stitching through time and showing itself amidst the fabric of all the daily goings-on. I see that love weaves together all things, that there is nothing of life that is not a part of the warp and woof, part of the stitching of love's handiwork. I say this, not as a belief, but more like a midwife present to the miracle and wonder of life, ready to receive the new promise, inchoate gift revealed—human being—word made flesh. It is, in fact, for me at the moment of birth, when one human being emerges from another, that I see most vividly the possibility that our lives are for one another. The very cry, the proclamation "I am" resounds and is held in the listening of the rest of the human family. At that moment one birth is all birth, one possibility all possibilities, one beginning all beginnings. We are here for life and we are here for one another, that is, to forward life and forward one another.

In this writing I do not use the word love frequently, and yet it is always that which moves me to give voice to the wonder of life, moves me to look continuously into the phenomenon of life and healing. Nothing that I say is sayable except that I am moved to include you in my life, to speak to you with dignity about that which I hold dear, to invite you to be in relationship with me as a fellow traveler, to accept your partnership, and in so doing, to create with you a home.

_____

Regarding the multitude of quotes —

To quote is to cite a passage, to make an opening, to bring something forward, to express a way of being, to bear witness . . .

> . . . so words
> guard the shape of man . . .
> even when man has fled and
> is no longer there.
>
> — George Seferis

It is a very personal act to find the speakings of other human beings, to listen the words-worlds of others. Poets, writers, philosophers, lovers of wisdom and life, return us to our source, to the dazzle of life itself. I have been gathering these quotes all my life. My life is spoken by them as a way of being in the ongoing speaking-listening of generations. The quotes are arranged in themes according to the chapters. Read them as Self speaking no matter how many or how diverse they seem. Read them as unspeakable speaking through words.

The stories of patients that illustrate this writing are factually accurate, except for the names, locales and individual traits which have been altered to protect privacy while preserving coherence.

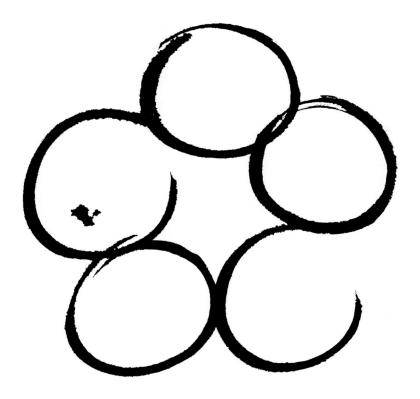

The daily round of movement
is where to look for the wonder of life . . .

Introduction

A book should be an axe that breaks the
frozen sea within us.

— Franz Kafka

Camerado, this is no book,
Who touches this touches a [person],
(Is it night? are we here together alone?)
It is I you hold and who holds you,
I spring from the pages into your arms . . . .

— Walt Whitman

This book is about healing. I dedicate my life to becoming masterful in the art of healing, the art of being alive. Traditional acupuncture is my training tool and my instrument for engaging with life—engaging with my own vital force, engaging this same impelling force of others.*

---

*The purpose of this healing art is to forward life—it is life medicine. Life is the essential force in being alive. It is that without which we are dead. Medicine is the art of healing. The word comes from the root "medeor" meaning heal, which also in Anglo-Saxon origin translates as whole (*haelan hal*). And so it is that I understand life medicine as the healing (wholing) art of being alive.

3

.... O pulse of my life!

O Thou transcendent,
Nameless, the fibre and the breath,
Light of the light, shedding forth universes, thou centre
  of them,
        . . . .
Thou pulse—thou motive of the stars, suns, systems,
That, circling, move in order, safe, harmonious,
Athwart the shapeless vastnesses of space,
How should I think, how breathe a single breath, how speak,
  if, out of myself,
I could not launch, to those, superior universes?

— Walt Whitman

The essential constituent of a human being is life, sometimes referred to as life force, Ch'i, élan vital, quickening
principle, *vis vitae*, breath of life, Promethean spark. How
we "know" this life force, this Ch'i, is through movement.
The Chinese observed the great movement of the Ch'i and
saw it as a journey of cycles. They spoke of these cycles as
the *Wu Hsing*, the five great changes, actions, motions of
nature. These actions become known as the Five Elements,
an interpretation of the movement of life as it manifests in
the seasons of the year and the seasons of a lifetime, as it
shows itself in every aspect of nature outside the human
being as well as within the course of human existence. All
movement, all actions, all changes are seen as the working of
the Ch'i as it cycles in the journey of the *Wu Hsing*. Nothing is
left out in the journey. Everything is considered a manifestation of life, of Ch'i, of the vital impulse. The daily round of
movement is where to look for the wonder of life.
All of this movement, the daily motion and emotion,
become the basis for the examination in traditional acupuncture. The practitioner explores the manifestations of the Ch'i
by asking, seeing, feeling, hearing the movement of the life
force. As practitioner and patient engage with the "show-

ings" of the Ch'i, they recognize the Life at the fundus of these manifestations; they heal; they come home; they are moved by life, consecrated to life and life's possibilities.

This is not a book about acupuncture. Acupuncture is not important in itself. No technology is. The data of techniques are fascinating, but not for the sake of themselves. They are important only insofar as they enable us to dive into the well of being, only insofar as they create access to being alive, only insofar as they support and forward our being home, our journey to ourselves. Ours is ". . . . the journey back to the Centre . . . . The return to the Centre is the journey home, back to the central hearth." (J. C. Cooper) Access to home, i.e., access to rest and peace, to harmony and balance, to an abiding centre where Being and being meet, where Self comes face to face with self—that is what any human endeavor is intent on furthering, the movement of Life in life on our way home.

In every body of technology is a vision of creation, and it is more or less hidden, more or less articulated. Inherent in the context of traditional acupuncture, in the body of information and interpretation, is a context for being alive, for healing. The context is a visionary design, a weaving together of what constitutes aliveness. What is the weave, the discourse for healing that acupuncture creates? Of what is the fabric called life according to this ancient tradition? What is the visionary design of this work?

In this writing, as in my first book, I intend to make available that vision—that is, the visionary design and the possibility for life that is inherent in acupuncture—not just for acupuncturists, students, patients, and health care practitioners, but for everyone engaged in being alive. ee cummings wrote that "love's function is to fabricate unknownness." This may be a perfect place to put that quote. This may also be a perfect place to put a quote from Dag Hammarskjöld:

Now. When I have overcome my fears—of others, of
myself, of the underlying darkness:
    at the frontier of the unheard-of.
    Here ends the known. But, from a source beyond it,
something fills my being with its possibilities.

It may be that in our exploration here together, we will
come close to the great mystery of healing, close to the fabric
of human being, close to a design for life. Perhaps we will
learn to fabricate one another in unknownness. Perhaps we
shall weave a whole out of our parts. Perhaps we shall wake
up as from a deep sleep to possibilities unheard-of.

"Camerado, this is no book . . . ."

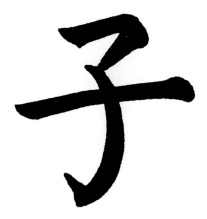

The Way To Do Is To Be

CHAPTER ONE

The Way To Do Is To Be

There is no need to run outside
For better seeing,
Nor to peer from a window. Rather abide
At the center of your being . . . .
Search your heart and see . . . .
The way to do is to be.

— Lao Tze

gateway of being: open your being, awaken,
learn then to be, begin to carve your face,
develop your elements, and keep your vision
keen to look at my face, as I at yours,
keen to look full at life right through to death,
faces of sea, of bread, of rock, of fountain,
the spring of origin which will dissolve our faces
in the nameless face, existence without face
the inexpressible presence of presences . . . .

— Octavio Paz

The Tao does nothing, yet nothing is left undone.

— Lao Tze

> The Greeks called "being" . . . . *parousia* . . . . The veritable
> translation would be a set or cluster of significations compris-
> ing "homestead, at-homeness, a standing in and by itself, a
> self-enclosedness, an integral presentness or thereness." . . . .
> it is to just this ground that we must strive to come home
> ("homecoming" is, as we shall see, both the process and the
> goal of authentic being).
>
>   — George Steiner

E verything comes forth from Being. Synonyms for
Being, that is, Being expressed in other words, are: essence,
existence, truth, prime constituent, vital principle, spirit,
quiddity, life, nature. Whatever I produce issues from my
being. "The ten thousand things are born of being." All of my
doings are predicated on my being. My actions are manifestations of being. Being is the constant in the process of life
itself. Doing is an accomplishment of being. "The way to do
is to be" points me homeward in my every activity, my every
deed, for what I intend to bring about must first be grounded
in my being. This is so no matter what arena of my humanity
I am operating in at any given moment, e.g., if I am to
achieve a powerful action in the treatment room I must stand
in my own life present to the truth of my life. The "doing" of
the treatment, then, becomes an expression of being. The
action of treatment becomes a response to the request of the
patient for guidance in a way of life harmonious to being
whole, to being Home in herself. In this context of being, in
the standing in the veracity of nature, doing is spontaneous,
effortless. My actions correlate freely and naturally with my
patient as we dive deep into the habitat of our being, of what
could be called the well of being.

In this dance of doing-being, the tale of the cook called
Ting is a superb illustration. Cook Ting is cutting up an ox for
Lord Hui of Wen, and his every movement is in concert with
his every other movement, likened to the "dance of the

mulberry grove." Lord Hui is moved by this excellence and inquires as to how skill can reach such perfection. Cook Ting lays his knife down and says: "That which I prize is Tao, and Tao goes beyond skill. When first I began to cut up an ox I saw only the ox itself. After three years I no longer saw the ox, and now it is through the spirit that I make my approach and not through the physical sight. Senses and understanding cease and the spirit takes over the action. I rely on the principles of nature, strike where there are great spaces, follow through the hidden openings, accept things as they are, never touching the ligaments and tendons, much less the main joints. There is no hacking. My knife has lasted nineteen years and has cut up several thousand oxen, and yet the blade is as if it had just left the whetstone. There is space between the joints and the knife-edge has no thickness. If what is without thickness enters where there is space, there is plenty of room." "How excellent," said the Lord of Wen, "by listening to the words of cook Ting I have learned to take care of my life."

"The spirit takes over the action" is another way of saying the being takes over the doing. "It is through the spirit that I make my approach" is a constituent of this man's mastery. His excellence and power as a butcher are derived from his essential being, his spirit. From there the "hidden openings" appear and the "great spaces" become his navigation tool. He does not hack and he does not cut. He is home with his action. The doer and the deed are one. He is the "dance of the mulberry grove," being and doing in perfect harmony. In this moment, in this mastery, all struggle and effort resolve. The Lord of Wen listens and in the listening openings and spaces "appear" from the cook's words giving rise to an amazing assertion from the Lord: "I have learned to take care of my life." Here is mastery begetting mastery, being begetting being, an act of healing, wholing, transformation, a following of the principles of nature. To take care of life is to be at home in life, present to our own being. Everything is an exercise in being, life present to life in the putting in of a needle, the plucking of a guitar string, the perceiving of a work of art, the peeling of an orange, the paying of a bill, the penetration of a lover, the pageantry of a pain. So be it. So be all of it. The great cosmic Doing is a hierophany of Being; humanity's endeavor is a sacred showing, hallowed manifestation for/to/of Life.

> Holy! Holy! Holy! Holy! Holy! Holy! Holy! Holy! Holy!
> Holy! Holy! Holy! Holy! Holy!
> The world is holy! The soul is holy! The skin is holy! The nose
> is holy! . . . .
> Everything is holy! everybody's holy! everywhere is holy! . . . .
> Holy forgiveness! mercy! charity! faith! Holy! Ours! bodies!
> suffering! magnanimity!
>
> — Allen Ginsberg

Infinite conversations open up from here: one is the seeming impossibility that "space" can come into view in something so ostensibly dense as the flesh of an ox. What is this phenomenon? Where must I be looking for an "opening" to appear? How must I be looking? Into what eyes and what ears can transformation show itself? Alan Watts noted that "the human body contains so much empty space that its ponderable elements could be condensed to the size of that very pinpoint, for its apparent solidity is an illusion arising from the rapid motion of its atomic components—as when a spinning propeller seems to become an impenetrable disk." What will it take for me to open up the illusion of density and closedness, to open to the diaphany of the physical world, the showing-through of openness? What is required of me to live life as an opening? to create openings? to see no obstructions? What does it take for me to "be" an opening? to be at one with all my actions? to be in perfect harmony, no hacking, no cutting, simply being present to the opening again and again and again and again?

What am I doing when I am doing acupuncture? Who am I being in the doing? Into what am I putting the needle? Into nothing, no thing, into space, an opening called human being? Into the earth of a heavenly being? Into the heaven of an earthly being? Are we all, as Rilke says, "Angels," beings in whom "the transformation of the visible into the invisible, which we are accomplishing, already appears in its completion . . . ."

A young woman named Jane is one of my patients. She came for treatment originally because a friend told her she could get some help for her painful menstruations and her struggles with food and weight. Those were her main complaints, the cause of her plaintive cries for support; yet when I asked her what she wanted more than anything else from treatment, she said, "I want my husband and my daughter to know how much I love them, how much their lives give me my life." She spoke as though she were "dawning," hearing herself give voice to the subsisting love and opening for life that she already is. She heard herself speak, and in her speaking I too could hear her promise to life. For Jane treatment has become a basic life support as she lives into her promise and grapples with daily issues, as she looks for the "openings" in life moment by moment. As for her symptoms, her periods are easier and she experiences herself as less moody. She struggles still with her weight, yet she has lightened up about food, enjoying it enough even to take up a gourmet cooking class. I have been treating her mostly via the Fire Element. She has much more access to life as joyful, as already accomplished. She lives from the home that she is for life. She is complete as is. She is a human being.

Another conversation generated from the chapter theme, "the way to do is to be," is an ongoing exploration of the question "What is required for mastery, for being present to life and accepting what is so?" There is a story from Chuang Tze to illustrate this conversation—it is the story of Old Camelback, who was a highly successful gardener. People wanted to know the secret of his success, but he denied having any particular method other than fostering natural tendencies, that is, forwarding life. He said, "In planting trees, be careful to set the roots straight, to smooth the earth around, to use good mould and to ram it down well. Then, don't touch the trees, don't think about them, don't go and look at them, but leave them alone to take care of themselves and nature will do the rest. I only avoid trying to make trees grow—others are forever running backwards and forwards to see how they are growing, sometimes scratching them to make sure they are still alive, or shaking them to see if they are sufficiently firm in the ground, thus constantly interfering with the natural bias of the tree and turning their affection and care into an absolute bane and curse. I only don't do these things. That's all."

Trusting in nature and encouraging what is natural constitute Old Camelback's success. He does not try. He simply doesn't do things to the trees. He does nothing. He gives them good birth, then lets them be, knowing the trees will grow themselves and be true to their own nature, thus making him a great gardener. To forward life requires trust, a recognition of partnership, a willingness to be at home with all living things, a commitment to the human conversation of stewardship, a seeing into the nature of everything.

Another question inherent in this conversation is the question of cause. I think it is fair to say that when something occurs we are always asking, How come? What caused it? Why? Yet even if we can get a "because," there is a further "why" and a further "because." We can ask for a long, long time what is the cause of sickness? And we can come up with causes. In fact, history is full of explanations for illness, rife with theories, and rampant with interpretations, stories of "How come?" ranging from the wrath of the gods to the promiscuity of germs, to the latest in advanced high-tech diagnoses, physical and psychological. We all have our interpretations. Acupuncture does too, and yet at the fundus of all the rationale, what we can say about sickness is that it *is*, or perhaps more accurately, *something* is and we call it *sickness*. We take it itself as a starting point. From there we begin an investigation, creating interpretations as we go to

14

enable us to say that the phenomenon we call sickness is open to continual knowing—and *unknowing.*

Another topic, I would say a gripping topic, around which big theories of cause grow is "healing." What causes it? What's the reason for it? Beyond all the possible explanations advanced so far, what *is* is that something occurs and we call it healing. It may be that all we can ever do is interpret and keep creating interpretations that enliven and empower us to engage in the phenomenon of healing, of sickness, of whatever life theme grips us. Like Socrates we can investigate the manifestations, the phenomena of life through what amount to unanswerable questions, knowing that we do not know, not knowing if we ever will know, yet willing to live into the inquiry which brings us ever alive to the phenomenon and all the inherent phenomena that life is. The Why?, How?, What caused it?, What's the reason for life itself? are superseded by the presence and possibility of life; and a question to gain entrance to presence and possibility may be not Why, but What, is life? What am I present to when what I call life is present?

I *be* in life. I *do* in life. Life is, at the least, paradox. It is unspeakable. Concepts will not bear it. It is our residence. Truth is at the heart of it. It *is* home. As T. S. Eliot says, "there is a lifetime burning in every moment" with the seeming impossibility of apprehending "the point of intersection of the timeless with time." Life is home. We dwell in life. All of the great questions in human history live here. We are arriving where we are and being home in the face of all circumstance, in the face of death, of life, of the intersections of survival and creation. Being is home. From my being comes my doing simply and easily, just in the process of life itself— Source eternally present, issuing forth continuously, epiphany of One in many.

And all is always now . . . .

— T. S. Eliot

Mother Ina Bergeron, a religious with whom I made a retreat, spoke of her twenty-seven-month imprisonment in China. During the confinement she was required to sit in one position with her head bowed, her hands on her lap, day in and day out. I imagine I would have gone crazy with the daily crushing realization of being imprisoned and not allowed to do anything. When I asked her how she managed, she told me: "Yes, yes, I wanted to do many things, but I could not. I began to see that life is not only doing. Life is being and I am free. Day after day I called on the Giver of Life to teach me to be."

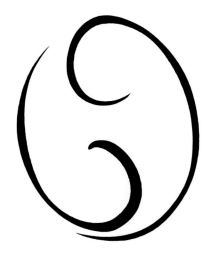

Home En Route

CHAPTER TWO

Home En Route

. . . . in the going I am there.

— Yevtushenko

YinYang . . . . the alternating pulse of the eternal series of surprises we call oneself.

— Chuang Tzu

I am heading home and I am already home. I am journeying in wholeness, dancing the duality of One, the YinYang
partnership. My world is made up of twos: on one hand, yet
on the other . . . . presence, absence . . . . ups and downs . . . .
fronts and backs . . . . tops and bottoms . . . . yes and no . . . .
being and becoming . . . . leaving and returning . . . . living
and dying . . . . you and me. Human life manifests in partnership from the very beginning as sperm and egg coming
together. One in two.

> He enters looking for her—searching past his brothers as
> she waits expectantly in the antechamber knowing that he is
> on his way. He finds her. She embraces him. They meet and
> are perfect for one another. The union destroys an old boun-
> dary and creates a new one. Neither knows where the other
> starts and stops. They become something they were not.
> They are a mystery, a completion of one another, a passion-
> ate mitosis as they travel together to a safe place—their
> lodging—their home. They grow together helping each form
> structures and internal powers—purposeful and detailed in
> their journey. Corded to their dwelling, they are safely con-
> nected, held and nourished, wandering freely within bounds
> of their anchor.
>
> And so they grow—fluid within fluid—a paradise of inti-
> mate communion and vast weaving—until they grow as big
> as their dwelling will allow. In the urgency of a greater call,
> wistful echoes of their first meeting are heard. It is time now.
> The next part of the journey beckons to them. Where they are
> they can go no further, and so, on the threshold of new life
> their old home holds them tight, hugs and squeezes and
> moves them lovingly and laboriously out of her with a power
> equal to their own. They are afraid. They are angry. They are
> eager and excited, expectant and joyous. They are sad. They
> feel for one another comforting and consoling. They find
> their route and in noble majesty they exit and enter in union.
> They crown as one. "All the Universe resounds with the
> joyful cry I am."*

*"The Story of a Sperm and Egg: YinYang Seeds of a Lifetime," by Dianne M.
Connelly, in the Spring 1981 *Journal of Traditional Acupuncture,* p. 17.

The human being is born into the swim of human experience and interpretation, into the continual interplay of one thing with another, into the dance of stories, cycles, rhythms, seasons, sounds, smells, tastes, touches, colors, emotions, into the constantly changing, unfolding, revolving, evolving life of other human beings—human beings all crying "I am" in as many voices as there are human beings. The one who has emerged from two enters a world in which she is already dependent on partnership for her very life. At least one other "I am" becomes her partner in the dance, or she dies. In the beginning the one she comes to call mother is her first partner. Home and mother are interchangeable. We human beings have left the insides of the mother to create a home outside her.

> To explore is to penetrate . . . . the world is the insides of the mother . . . .
>
> — Norman O. Brown

We have moved from belly to arms and lie flesh against flesh, still at home, yet distinct as two. This begins our dance of duality, our two-part harmony, our duet of self and other. We are not always one with her now. She does not take us with her everywhere. She is not always present. I cry and I cry for her. I do not know how to be with her absence. If she is my home and she is gone, where am I? Where is home? I begin my search, this human being's quest for home.

> All interpretation is to conquer a remoteness, a distance . . . .
>
> — Paul Ricoeur

Consciousness, they say, begins with distance, with a baby's new sense of separateness from the world, and pain in our remoteness from the objects of desire. Beyond the close boundaries of our own small bodies the universe spins away, and we start trying to understand it; to go home again. In fact, we have just created that home by our very distance from it,

without which it—the center—would not exist. "The home
that is nowhere, that is the true home," said a Chinese adept.

— Thomas Buckley

In one of my children's books called *Are You My Mother?*
by P. D. Eastman, a baby bird comes out of its egg. In the
meantime mama bird has gone to get some food for baby.
Baby looks all over asking "Where is my mother?", falls out
of his tree and begins the search for his mama. He goes to a
kitten, a hen, a dog, a cow, a boat, a plane and a big machine
he calls a "snort," asking each in turn "Are you my mother?"
"Where am I?" said the baby bird. "I want to go home! I
want my mother!" Eventually, eventually he finds her and,
in finding her, he is home.

We are homesick for ourselves and for each other. As we
enter the great human company at the moment of birth the
world of humanity becomes my home first represented by
the one I call mother. She is my first partner in my life's
journey. In her presence I am home. In her absence I am
wanderer. I seek and seek her everywhere. I am homesick
for her and for myself. With her partnership I explore the
world, and greet creation.

This conversation is not intended as a paean to mother, yet
it is a hymn to life and how life manifests in partnership,
whatever that partnership be: parent-child, lover-beloved,
friend-friend, husband-wife, sister-brother, teacher-student,
patient-practitioner, employee-employer, self-other. Partnership is the basis for all relationship. We have no existence
apart from one another. You are the world for me, and I for
you.

We are the world. We are home for each other. We move
between certainty and uncertainty, valleys and peaks, hard
patches and easy patches, storms and calms, befores and
afters, comings and goings, always home.

One depends on two to illuminate it, just as two depend on
one for their meaning. One and two do not alter one another.

They exhibit and express each other. The unity of life is never altered. This dance turns up everywhere, beginning at the first moments of movement from womb-woman to womb-world. As a fruit of the womb of woman, I am delivered already dancing, already the dance. My heart beats. My breath comes and goes. My "I" is distinguished from those who birthed me. We are separate, yet I am recognized as human. I cry. The force of life exhibits itself in my flailings. I am life. I am life with no categories. I am at the centre of human being, a being at home exploring the contours of this new "world" dwelling. I am the world, all-encompassing, enfolding. Then, I begin to make boundaries, draw distinctions, create otherness and forget that all of it is home, that I am home. To speak and to share I create categories which in combination give a composite expression of home. I begin to see that I make my world up of twos as a way of speaking about life, as a way of speaking about the goings-on at home. "Twoness" gives partnership which opens up the possibility of union. In my oneness, my integer, arises a squawking for "other," a call from my integrity that demands responses to the call.

> As he hastens between them (Yin and Yang), the pilgrim unites the two poles within himself. Duality, which is the source of all movement and all phenomena, must constantly return—or be returned—to Unity, its origin and its end.
>
> — Gai Eaton

My struggle and my strength arise from the same source, and exhibit one another. The world that I am summons me to make room for the expression of the whole, for every realm of human experience, for the one and the many. If healing is about being whole, then every expression of being wants acknowledgment, including the things I don't like. Most of us hide out, and where we hide out is in the thought that if we did not hide we would not be acceptable, that there are parts of me that do not belong in the whole, parts that are not an expression of being in the womb-world. Our illnesses are born and bred on not recognizing ourselves, on not seeing that we are always already home while en route. If we are willing to take another human being with us to our secret places, to the places where we deny or do not recognize ourselves, then in the moment of arriving to our "secret" we enter ourselves newly. The person we allow to come with us, the intimate traveling companion, comes without adding anything or taking anything away, comes silently, empty and following exactly. The healing is the discovery of the self. It is the homecoming, the returning home, the restoring of all lost parts.

> All things come home at eventide,
> like birds that weary of their roaming.
> And I will hasten to thy side, ... Homing.
>
> — Old English Song

As I am writing this I experience what I call excitement and joy, excitement and joy in the face of homing. In a day's time I am lost and found over and over again. Forgetting and recalling myself over and over. The kingdom of illness is designed on a pattern of forgetting, a forgetting that has gotten stuck, a forgetting that seems to have no re-membering, a forgetting that would have us be lost to ourselves, a forgetfulness of being. So, if I take you to my forgetting, to my sickness, and you bring your self as guide, as coach, as practitioner, once more I come home, and see that I have been home all along, and that my illness has been instrumental in leading me there one more time. I interpret the everlasting comings and goings of the dance of life, the alternating forgettings and rememberings, the endless agonies and ecstasies of daily life. The story of the Taoist farmer illustrates a way of interpreting the dance of life's events:

The farmer's horse ran away. That evening the neighbors gathered to commiserate with him since this was such bad luck. He said, "May be." The next day the horse returned, but brought with it six wild horses, and the neighbors came exclaiming at his good fortune. He said, "May be." And then, the following day, his son tried to saddle and ride one of the wild horses, was thrown, and broke his leg. Again the neighbors came to offer their sympathy for his misfortune. He said, "May be." The day after that, conscription officers came to the village to seize young men for the army, but because of the broken leg the farmer's son was rejected. When the neighbors came in to say how fortunately everything had turned out, he said, "May be."

— Lieh Tze, as told by Alan Watts

Home is all embracing, a continuous inclusion of all events: this too and this too and this too and this too. Home en route. Home is the place from which I have come and to which I return. Home is where I always am. All circumstances call me to new steps in the dance. All sickness points me there. All sickness is homesickness. All healing is homecoming. Sharing moves me homeward.

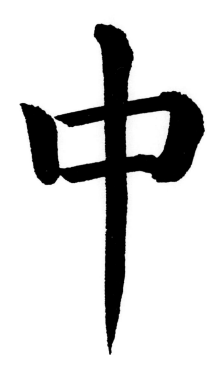

The Practice Of Being Home

CHAPTER THREE

The Practice Of Being Home

(To teachers, i.e., practitioners)

In You, whoe'er you are, my book perusing,
In I myself—in all the World—these ripples flow,
All, all, toward the mystic Ocean tending.

— Walt Whitman

Our knowledge that we shall not pass this way again—
almost unbearable—although it makes
each moment precious in itself,
strikes even deeper if we come to feel
the signs and patterns of the mystical
on every tree and bush and turning wheel.

— Dick Allen

As we live, we are transmitters of life.
. . . .
Give, and it shall be given unto you
is still the truth about life.
. . . .
It means kindling the life-quality where it was not,
even if it's only in the whiteness of a washed pocket-
    handkerchief

> — D. H. Lawrence

Not *how* the world is, is the mystical, but that it is.

> — Ludwig Wittgenstein

This chapter, "The Practice of Being Home," is at the heart of this whole book. The practice of being home is the action of the mystic, the bringing of the mystical into the realm of everyday activities—not mystical as mysterious, but mystical as daily awe-inspiring; mystical as fundamental in the moment to moment universe; mystical as the only possible context to hold the whole, given the multitudinous manifestations that comprise it. The mystical lives in the field of daily action, the training ground of all creature activity. "In our era, the road to holiness necessarily passes through the world of action." (Dag Hammarskjöld) Without daily action, without the living in the "unbearable precious," our life becomes merely a belief and a study, not a living and being alive and in awe, except in rare moments in which we can do no other.

The treatment room and all that is brought to bear there, all of the magnificent, simple tools of diagnosis—the askings and listenings and seeings and touchings—are all reachings-in to the human being; they reach beyond life as a study, to life as the very field of action of One, of the Mystical, no matter what the symptom or the reason the person has come for treatment. The practitioner-mystic does not stop to question the bounds of her own or her patient's ordinariness or extraordinariness. Rather, following the words of Chuang Tze ("Leap into the boundless and make it your home."), she leaps into the boundless with her patient and together they make it their home. Likewise, though speaking from a different tradition, St. Basil says: "The human person is a creature that has received the commandment to become God." The treatment room is our daily invitation to creation. It is an ongoing call into existence through, with, and beyond all the present conditions and circumstances.

In being alive and in awe, the practitioner-mystic is in love with the One, the Integrity inherent in all she finds in the field that is her own life, her patient's life and all life. She summons us to take part in evolution, to give our attention to creating life, to returning to the origin of everything, to returning ourselves to creation, to exploring the original inspiration.

The practice of being home is the practice of living paradox, being human yet commanded to be God, being bounded yet summoned to leap into the boundless, kindling life-quality in every action be it grand or humble, living the Way of the Tao by not doing anything in particular, being separate and at one with the entire creation.

> One day when I was feeling like a motherless child, which I was, it come to me: that feeling of being part of everything, not separate at all. I knew that if I cut a tree, my arm would bleed. And I laughed and I cried and I run all round the house. I knew just what it was. In fact, when it happen, you can't miss it.
>
> — Shug, in Alice Walker's *The Color Purple*

The same paradox of living, the paradox of the mystical, is referred to by T. S. Eliot in "Burnt Norton":

> The dance along the artery
> The circulation of the lymph
> Are figured in the drift of stars . . . .

What courses through us courses through all of nature, that is, the perpetual movement of life. "Attention to nature is life in action." (Ortega y Gasset) We fall endlessly into ourselves action after action regardless of the particular room of human activity—the classroom, livingroom, boardroom, bathroom, bar room, guest room, family room, bedroom, music room, treatment room. We are with ourselves wherever we go, not even aware of how much life is living us, gripping and training us, how much we are one with all else, how much every symptom houses a life theme found not just there in the symptom's plaintive cry.

The theme of the mystic is always and everywhere potently available. I am reminded of the kid in the movie *The Karate Kid*. His daily discipline houses the very abstractions of karate that he espouses and he does not see that this is so until he is called into action. At the moment the teacher confronts him, the boy is astonished to see that he is already home, already accomplished. He has been learning by living, by following the instruction of the one he has chosen as guide, teacher, coach. The paradox of practice is the paradox that all is in all, that the flow of life is evidenced in everything and in nothing in particular, in the guest house of the mystic, the whiteness of a washed pocket handkerchief, in all the events of the whole day long. The practice of being home is an ongoing kindling of the life quality. It is the practice of finding our way home in every moment, every condition, every symptom and every circumstance. It is the continuous underbelly of being human. It is the place of the mystic. The practice of being home *is* being home.

> Who ever reads me will be in the thick of the scrimmage, and if he doesn't like it—if he wants a safe seat in the audience— let him read somebody else . . . .
>
> — D. H. Lawrence

There is no "safe seat in the audience." What we are addressing here is the adventure of being alive, the being in the "thick of the scrimmage" at all times. There is no respite from life, no stopping. There is peace and stillness possible only in the heart of the action. Storm and turbulence are daily fare too. There is no security. We are always at risk.

> Security is mostly a superstition. It does not exist in nature, nor do the children of men as a whole experience it. Avoiding danger is no safer in the long run than outright exposure. Life is either a daring adventure, or nothing.

> — Helen Keller

Circumstances would not in themselves be cause for knowing we are home. In the midst of daily perturbations we are hard pressed to practice being home, hard pressed to "see" that all expressions of life, including the tumult, the wrangles, the irritants, are the field of the mystical, are the expressions of One. In the "thick of the scrimmage" it is often hard for us, the players, to remember what we are doing here, hard to get in the presence of life. Coaching, then, becomes crucial to a player committed to the conscious moment-to-moment taking on of life. Coaching becomes the wake-up call from one whose vision of the possibilities of the game is a match for the greatness of the player.

To the practitioner-coach, the patient is a player in the heart of the scrimmage of her own life, committed to taking her life on. The same is true for the teacher: the student is the chief protagonist for her own life. The teacher becomes coach in the adventure of the student's life, just as for the patient, the practitioner becomes coach for the patient's life. The coaches also have coaches, their teachers and practitioners, their mentors of the mystical, who assist them in the practice of being home, of taking on their lives in every possible way. And, in turn, the patients and students become coaches for others to be home. When I treat one person, another family member will thank me for the new life she, and often the whole family experiences, as a result of that one person's homecoming. I see that as one family member "arrives" she becomes the occasion of arrival for the entire family. She ushers them all home. And then they too act as life support for everyone around them. In this way treatment is public. People become guides for the lives of those around them. I envision concentric circles of creation, human being to human being, the heart of the mystic to the heart of the mystic, giving life. This is how life grows: one person influencing another. It is certainly how a practice grows.

Now, let's speak of one we would call teacher, coach, guide, mystic—that is, practitioner—and the action we would call teaching, coaching, guiding, awe-inspiring—that is, practicing. It is fitting to have this topic as part of the chapter on "The Practice of Being Home," fitting because we are addressing all practice, not just my practice which is traditional acupuncture. The specific practice, the specific line of life action, be it medicine, history, football, parenting, writing—all human endeavor—requires us to be living in residence with ourselves using every event and every person to teach, coach, guide and inspire. In our training program at the Traditional Acupuncture Institute, though the content is traditional acupuncture, the context is human homing. I suggest that all practice of anything has humanity being at home with itself as its underlying intent, its context, its living philosophy—and humanity being at home with itself is awesome. Without awe, astonishment, breathtaking wonder, life withers and dies while we are still alive. Without awe we are not at home.

"Astonishment is the beginning of philosophy" is an assertion of many philosophers, including Plato, Aristotle, and Heidegger.

> Live in a perpetual great astonishment.
>
> — Theodore Roethke

Late on the third day, at the very moment when, at sunset, we were making our way through a herd of hippopotamuses, there flashed upon my mind, unforeseen and unsought, the phrase, "Reverence for Life."

— Albert Schweitzer

The highest point a man can attain is not knowledge . . . . but something even greater, more heroic . . . . Sacred Awe!

— Nikos Kazantzakis

. . . . You are not here to verify,
Instruct yourself, or inform curiosity
Or carry report. You are here to kneel
Where prayer has been valid. And prayer is more
Than an order of words . . . .

— T. S. Eliot

Explanation separates us from astonishment, which is the only gateway to the incomprehensible.

— Eugene Ionesco

A teacher creates worlds. Each world created is a sacred vessel. As Roethke defines the word, "Teacher: one who carries on her education in public." She creates by giving voice and giving silence, by speaking words and listening from whence the words come. She can not be teacher-coach-awe-inspirer without giving herself away, without opening to her own astonishing aliveness, without publicly wondering and wandering in her own beginner's mind.

"Don't say: create." These words from Roethke express the promise of one's life as teacher. Life is awesome, awe-filled. She teaches from awe, and not from her opinions, beliefs, advice. She does whatever will forward the life of the one or ones she is coaching. "Teach as an old fishing guide takes out a beginner." (Roethke) She lives at the edge of life as a creative act, continuous and evolving, not infrequently terrified of her own godliness; not infrequently enraptured by the joy and fun of it all; always grappling with her own humanity. "When you discard arrogance, complexity, and a few other things that get in the way, sooner or later you will discover that simple, childlike, and mysterious secret known to those of the Uncarved Block: Life is Fun." (Benjamin Hoff, *The Tao of Pooh*)

She provides a compelling invitation, an urgency to all her listeners to open now in this moment, here in this place, not some other day, some other where. This is the holy moment, the holy place, the holy you. Three classical imperative questions provoke us: If not now, then when? If not here, then where? If not you, then who? The teacher-coach calls us home again and again and again to this is it, life is now, right here, through me, through you, and not just where our skin begins and ends. She urges us to live doing everything for the last time. The teacher summons us to remind each other of the unconditional holiness, wholeness, intactness of our lives, and of life itself. She insists that we teach by giving ourselves, our history, our knowings, our seeings and listenings away. The teacher imparts a body of distinctions to empower the student to live, and to live not so much by helping, but by giving herself away. "Give a person a fish—he eats for a day. Teach a person to fish—he eats for a life time."

> There are times when it becomes impossible for me to teach. No matter where I look I see only God, wearing so many masks, playing in so many forms. Who is the teacher then? Who is to be taught?
>
> — Swami Prabhavanda

For the teacher-coach-practitioner, life manifests as dance, as walking the circle in daily steps familiar and unfamiliar. The coach is the creator of context for the entire dance, for all the steps. She is not "stuck" on any one way. She knows she has no answer to give. She also knows that as teacher she is student, learning to be home herself in all the domains of her life. Homing is wanted everywhere. She is a protagonist for life, an antagonist for anything other. The teacher-mystic is an inquirer, an instigator of inspiration, committed to aliveness—this is so regardless of the content to be taught, or the material to be covered. What we "know" always derives from unknowing, that is, from standing open to life's phenomena, open to the "ten thousand things." The teacher-poet Theodore Roethke says: "All knowledge lives in paradox," and "All roads lead to the self . . . ." Behind every knowing is the thrust of life itself as we human beings reach to embrace it and in many instances reach to capture it, that is, to capture ourselves. Teacher, like a maestro, conducts us through every knowing, through every piece of music, back to music itself, to life itself, from whence we come. Life transparently grounds every knowing, every subject, every teaching. Teacher calls us awake beyond the readily apparent and points us all, including herself, homeward.

Henri Bergson, a philosopher of history, addresses this theme, this practice of being home, though in different words in the following passage:

> The soul of the great mystic does not come to a halt at the [mystical] ecstasy as though that were the goal of a journey . . . . The great mystic has felt the truth flow into him from its source like a force in action . . . . His desire is with God's help to complete the creation of the human species . . . . The mystic's direction is the very direction of the "elan" of life. It is that "elan" itself, communicated in its entirety to privileged human beings whose desire it is thereafter to set the imprint of it upon the whole of mankind . . . .

To practice is to put into action. To practice being home is to put home into action. It is the practice of the mystic to be home and bring awe to the day, every day, simply being in the presence of life itself. The home of the mystic is the realm of the teacher-practitioner, the kingdom of human being. The practice of being home—here, now, as is, at one—is an ongoing way of being a human being.

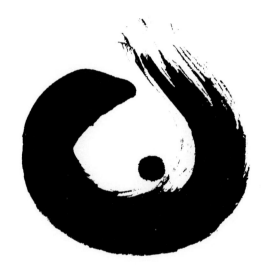

Homing

CHAPTER FOUR

Homing

(the act of going home or of coming home,
homeward bound)

Home is where we start from . . .

— T. S. Eliot

"Warren," she said, "he has come home to die:
You needn't be afraid he'll leave you this time."

"Home," he mocked gently.

"Yes, what else but home?
It all depends on what you mean by home.
Of course, he's nothing to us, any more
Than was the hound that came as a stranger to us
Out of the woods, worn out upon the trail.

"Home is the place where, when you have to go there,
They have to take you in."

— Robert Frost

How do I know about the world? By what is within me.

— Lao Tze

Nowhere, Beloved, will world be but within us—Our life passes in transformation.

— Rainer Maria Rilke

The immediate service of all human beings is necessary simply because the only way to find God is to see him in his creation and to be one with it . . . . I know that I cannot find him apart from my own humanity.

— Mahatma Gandhi

. . . he's a human being . . . . attention must be paid.

— Arthur Miller

The movement of the Tao consists in Returning . . . .

— Lao Tze

This ancient system of healing—traditional acupuncture—a human system having been carried and delivered to all the rest of us by the Chinese, addresses the nature of us, individually and collectively. We are seen to be between heaven and earth, balancing the Elements, simultaneously guided by and leading the evolutionary and infinite abilities of life. We watch the trees and in the simplicity of seeing, that which we call "tree" in all its variations comes into being. All are accounted for with not one left out. In the observation of its life, every tree has value and standing in its own right.

Like ourselves, a tree is one and many. Its roots speak of all roots. Its earth-boundness is all earth-boundness. Its branches and foliage and fruits are all reachings and manifestations and produce. Like a tree we are who we are in a singular integrity and proclaim to every other one of us the possibility that is each uniqueness. We need only to look at the nature of the phenomenon we are in order to see those possibilities.

As we investigate we begin to see as the Chinese farmer sees, the profound relationships within nature, relationships that in the seeing shape our very lives. A simple example of this is in the creation of a garden. Creating a garden depends on a balance of the elements of nature and unless I pay attention to the interactions of the elements, their interdependence and impact on one another, I can not create a garden. The earth will hold and germinate seeds only when its relationship to the sun and rain and mineral is in a harmonious balance. So I shape my creation upon my observation of how nature works, that is, in balance and harmony of all things.

Likewise for the creation of the "garden" I am, I need look to the Nature of who I am. I must see how I work with all my parts engaged and in balance with one another. Within the tradition of Oriental medicine from which acupuncture derives, are the makings of a powerful conversation about who human beings are. Lao Tze says that how we know about the world is by what is within us. If that is so, then part of the conversation of Oriental medicine addresses the question, What is within us?, which leads us into discussions about how we function, and what are our functions. I want here to replace the word "function" with "calling." However, I also want to give it the dictionary definition of "specific power of acting" one's "appropriate part," coming from the Latin verb *fungi* meaning to execute, i.e., to complete, accomplish, bring forth, carry out. We are continually making interpretations about our daily functions, our daily callings—the carrying out and completing of each day. But, what is it really, in a day's time that I am called to? And, in beginning to observe these functions will I start to see the nature of the garden that is Dianne? Will I open to the balance of, the dance of, what is within me? In this paragraph I am seeing how the poet Rilke has served me in his invitation: "learn to live the questions . . . . " The conversation that Oriental medicine opens is full of liveable questions.

So from here I enter the conversation—what am I called to in a day's time? What are the observations I can make regarding my own nature? And, then, as we go we may begin to see some possibilities past our up-til-now seeing.

This morning I awakened to the sun, full shining on my face. For a moment the gift of light and warmth held me captive. There was nothing else. Every sense, every thought, every mood gone and I dwelled in present time, alive and awake. Life, diaphanous in such a moment, asserted itself and I no longer made any distinctions of separateness, distinctions which at other times seem inevitable and essential. Life took me. So, the day opens with a quest—where will I place my boundaries today? Do I end where my skin does? Who is "I"? Clearly, a being in a question is a being open to looking at the nature of life, and willing to see it whole and as gift with no boundaries. If I had not an opening I could not even ask the questions.

A question is already a looking beyond what I presently know or have access to. This is particularly important when a patient comes in for treatment holding herself as a person who is stuck, who has no room to move, or no question from which to see life as gift. She is bound to her symptom with no opening, yet the very action of seeking help—even if it is held that an "expert" will tell her what to do—is a reaching beyond a known to some other possibility. The symptom is a breakdown in which she holds herself as not having certain possibilities, yet it is only because she can see some possibility of an opening that she is even in breakdown. "Indeed, the hidden and the manifest give birth to each other . . . . high and low set measure to each other . . . . " (Lao Tze) We only make the distinction breakdown in light of breakthrough.

What manifests is symptom. What manifests as hidden is well-being, that is, the well of being from which the symptom is born.

For the most part in this Western culture we hold our symptoms as opposed to our health. They are problems to be gotten rid of, not an expression of our health. They are "bad" and produce an experience of upset, also interpreted as pain. They are to be fought, not embraced. The context for symptom is generally one of hostility and fear, a "bigger-than-I-am," "how-did-this-happen-to-me" circumstance, a being a victim of some mysterious happening beyond my personal ken to deal with. The usual stance with a symptom is one of "I am sick, and this is evidence of that," rather than "I am well, and in the midst of my wellness I have a struggle that is expressed in this symptom." Our relationships to our symptoms are debilitating and disempowering to ourselves. Notice, I am speaking about our relationships to our symptoms, that is, how we bring ourselves to them. I see that with our symptoms, our ills, our pains, we create not healing relationships, but rather battles, even full-scale war attempting to survive, to "kill" our symptoms so we will not die. For the most part, our conversations with our symptoms are fights, and so our victories turn out clever, but not very powerful or creative. Perhaps an appropriate question here is, what is possible?

Two thoughts come to mind that seem at first to be disconnected. One is the work of Carol Gilligan whose book *In a Different Voice* calls us to look at the planet now and what may be possible for us as a human family. She notes the possibilities in examples such as this one: When shown a picture of a battlefield, little boys are likely to ask, Who won?, whereas shown the same battlefield, little girls are likely to ask, What about the mommy of the boy who was hurt?

The other thought is from the sermons of John Donne: "Tribulation is treasure in the nature of it, but it is not current money in the use of it, except we get nearer and nearer our home . . . ."

How do these thoughts connect with our looking at symptom? For me they are thoughts that engender a not-so-usual interpretation of symptom based on relationship and purposefuless. At any moment we can ask the questions of survival, or the questions of relationship: Who won?, and what about her, what about him? This is a time in the global village and in our personal selves to be engaged in empowering conversations. We are shifting the context of life with each other from you or me to you and me. We are shifting the context of health from you or the symptom to you and the symptom. We become the room in which the symptom takes place, rather than the position opposite the symptom, that is, opposition. I daresay that if we viewed in slow motion a scene from a battlefield from any era, and took away the weapons, what we would see would be human beings reaching for one another, trying to "get" one another, trying to make an impact, a connection, a difference.

Donne's "tribulation is treasure in the nature of it . . . ." is powerfully congruent with the Oriental notion that our struggle and our strength emerge from the same source, and that were we to follow either to the ends of being we would find ourselves at home. Is it possible then, to open to our symptoms in such a way that we begin to find our way home, no matter how lost we have been, or how circuitous the route has seemed? Is there an unaddressed expression of creation inchoate in the symptom? Does the irritant summon us to our source?

Have we been overlooking a wondrous human power to create symptoms as a call to come home, to ourselves and to each other? What if, like the story of the prodigal son, we have left home, journeyed along different paths, had different symptoms and circumstances as guides leading us home again, to the home that has always been there, home immanent en route. What if, hidden in our symptoms were all the signposts and mapping we needed in order to be at home? Would that not shift our "tribulations," shift our entire relationship to our symptoms, our health, our medical care system?

I considered calling this book *Taking Down the Treatment Room Walls* because I find that what takes place in the treatment room is what we would have take place everywhere in every room, that is, an adventure, a quest, an expedition into self no matter where or what the self is experiencing or presenting. An old British definition of "quest" is "to bay on the trail of," bay as with a "deep bark or cry, as of dogs in hunting," bay so as to "drive or bring to a stand in the chase." Another definition of "quest" is "to search or seek for; inquire into, ... seek or follow a trail . . . ." One of the great diagnostic tools in Oriental medicine is "to ask," and its correlate diagnostic tool is "to listen." The "To ask" is the "baying on the trail" of another human being the likes of which exists nowhere else on the planet. The exact identity of this one person is nowhere to be found except right there in the room. She is her own identification and so her expression of herself in her words, her symptoms, her presence, is the place to look for her, the place to inquire into the nature of this human being, the place to find her and therefore to "bring her to a stand" for herself. As Francis Thompson says in his poem "The Hound of Heaven":

> I fled Him, down the nights and down the days;
> I fled Him down the arches of the years;
> I fled Him, down the labyrinthine ways
>   Of my own mind; and in the mist of tears
> I hid from Him, and under running laughter.
> Up vistaed hopes I sped;
> And shot, precipitated,
> Adown Titanic glooms of chasmed fears,
> From those strong Feet that followed, followed after.
> But with unhurrying chase,
> And unperturbed pace,
> Deliberate speed, majestic instancy,
> They beat—and a Voice beat
> More instant than the Feet—
> "All things betray thee, who betrayest Me . . . ."

The person in the treatment room is unique in all the world. Her very being is the territory of the quest. She is whom she is seeking. Her presence there is itself an inquiry into who she is and an invitation to the practitioner, her chosen fellow traveler, to "bay on her trail," to inquire with her into the phenomenon of her life, the "chase" of her days and nights into the labyrinthine ways she has come to know. And so we go, practitioner and patient, into the realm of this human being seeking the nature of her, bringing her to a stand for herself.

And is this not what each of us, no matter who we are or what room we are in, want from each other, that is, a listening to the cry that our life is, so that we are not alone in our journey? Maybe we are already on each other's trails and lost paths. Maybe we are already.

I have always been taken by the power of great poetry, especially great love poetry. In the addressing of the beloved, or the speaking about the beloved the words of the poet call forth something holy, and in the reading I become the beloved, the holy one, as though I am not only included in the poem, but am the source and subject of it. At the moment of reading, god-being and human-being are interchangeable.

Now, what does this have to do with the treatment room? Poetry, according to ee cummings "is being, not doing. If you wish to follow, even at a distance, the poet's calling . . . . you've got to come out of the measurable doing universe into the immeasurable house of being." To me, this has everything to do with the treatment room, for my relationship with my patient is in the realm of her being, and though I care how she "does" her life, I deeply care about how she "be" in the doing of her life. As she and I look together into her life addressing the this and thats—for example, her relationship with food, with sleep, with what brought her there in the first place and really with all the aspects of her aliveness—together we begin to be a kind of poetry. We are two human beings together calling forth the nature of the beloved, the holy, examining the "stuff" of life and finding there a god in "the immeasurable house of being." I mean this in a most profound way. It is, for me, the wonder and the privilege of being a practitioner, that is, being present when the god of human being, and just as accurately, when the human being of god, shows up. And in the nature of this work is a call to aliveness beyond even what we have so far imagined as possible for us human beings. The content of our lives—the symptoms, the circumstances, the daily goings-on, the "stuff"—takes on a whole new context when examined as expressions of being. What a wondrous phenomenon, the phenomenon of human being.

The other day one of my patients gave me a gift, and before she gave it to me she said: "Dianne, this is for you and it is for all the students you teach and other patients you see." She then told me the following story: "Yesterday," she said, "I met a fat, red-haired woman with freckles and very fat feet. Now, this may sound silly but I want you to know how much I hate fat feet, really hate fat feet, and this woman had really fat feet. Yet, I could see this woman as godly. Before our work together, there is no way this woman would have been god to me. I would not have been able to see her, really see her. I have had no room for her—and me. Dianne, thank you for working with me here in this room exactly as I am. I am coming home. Thank you."

I have entitled this book _All Sickness is Homesickness._ Homesickness is a yearning to be home in one's self. It is not a private matter. One's self includes others. The work of Oriental medicine, indeed, of any healing art, is to open a conversation for being well, that is, being at home. Healing, wholing, transformation is a public matter. Acupuncture supports a person to create a powerful context for healing as is, no matter what. Within that context, anything can come up, any symptom, any story, any struggle, any strength. There is room for everything and everyone, no matter who we are or what's going on. There is no way we have to be. We can be who we are and open to the possibilities of life. The contribution of this five-thousand-year-old conversation and interpretation to our modern western-world conversation and interpretation is, in the words of a colleague, "a great and humbling gift that invites us to exclaim at every moment . . . . God, You came like this, too!' "

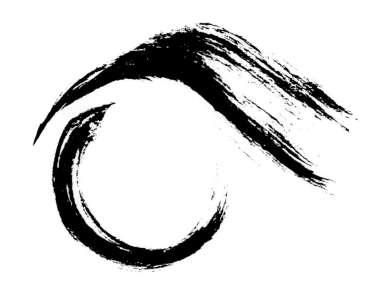

The Way Home

CHAPTER FIVE

The Way Home

A journey of a thousand leagues starts from
where your feet stand.

— Lao Tze

. . . . recurring in this body, bears you home . . . .

— James Dickey

Hence, only he who is willing to give his body for
the sake of the world is fit to be entrusted
with the world.
Only he who can do it with love is worthy of being
the steward of the world.

— Lao Tze

All attitudes, all the shapeliness, all the
      belongings of my or your body or of
      anyone's body, male or female,
      . . . .
The exquisite realization of health;
O I say these are not the parts and poems of
      the body only, but of the soul,
O I say now these are the soul!

                      — Walt Whitman

I look up the word "way" and find other words like thoroughfare, throughway, route, passage, journey. Then I look up those words and find main road, passage free from obstruction, all-embracing journey. Each word leads me on to another and another. Each word gives expression to another facet of that for which I look. Each word opens to something else until I begin to see that a simple little quest for the meaning of a word is opening me to the entire world of human interpretation, and that I can get any place I have to go right from here. In fact, I see that I can only get someplace from here. Here is where I start, here where my "feet stand." Where I am heading is into the meanings of life created by us human beings as we interact with each other through our words. We are making up meanings and creating paths out of them to lead us in and out of each other's lives. When I take up one word I am taking up the entire universe. When I take up one word I am taking up the creation. When I take up one word I am taking up the Word. With one word we are on our way home. We are in communication, sharing Life.

It's very seductive to write as though I have answers and am giving them to you. I don't. If I did, you might come away from this interaction thinking some new things. I would like that, but it is not what this exploration is intended for. There's something more powerful than that for us, something more akin to creating together, something more like seriously traveling together in life. I can tell you the bits I think I know. You can tell me the bits you think you know. Yet, neither of us knows what we do not know. We may not even know what it is to journey together, what it is to give to each other the life born of our days. Do we know to free our passage from obstruction, to complete each other throughout the whole from beginning to end, to see each other through, to take the road home?

This word "way" enters us into the conversation of voyage, travel, journey. It also gives entrance to the conversation of self and other, e.g. my way, your way, their way, the way, a way. Furthermore, it gives rise to the question Where? *Quo Vadis?* Whither does the journey take us? Are we all in this together? Are all of us, no one missing, fellow travelers? Where are we going? From whence have we come? Where are we now? How do we get where we are not?

I use the words "coming home" as a way of speaking of the journey. Others might say returning to source, undertaking the whole, knowing the self, being at one, living the moment sacred, creating the vision, interpreting the divine, seeing unity everywhere, loving life as is, listening godliness, restoring to nature. All of these are expressions of arrival, of being present to our own lives, of living at home, being one with the journey. The journey is home. Life is home, and life is voyaging in Self. We are never not home, never not in life, never not journeying.

Our vehicles of transport for the journey are our bodies. We are incorporated. We are beings clothed in flesh; embodied in bone, muscle, sinew, blood; incarnate life— pulsating corpus with openings for entry and exit, for participating in the world of human existence. The body is a privileged route in the engagement with the mystery of being, of healing, of being home in ourselves. Transformation is an ongoing creation of our corporeal being. Every bodily function is an amazing phenomenon, continuously in action moving from one form to another, one state to another, one motion to another. Every cell is voyaging— climbing, trekking, turning, tumbling, passing, splitting, coursing, generating, coming, going, changing, absorbing, dying—voyaging the internal valleys, caverns, rivers, peaks, at home in the cosmos incarnate.

The invitation on the way home is to enter the places that we think we know, newly, and to admit our own lostness. In so many ways I do not know my body, my incarnation, my being clothed in flesh, my dwelling. Being present to my body, to the workings of my corpus requires a shift from a ho-hum-so-what to an amazement and wonder. It requires dwelling-thinking. My most personal and wonder-filled experiences of body have been the pregnancies and births of my children. Never before had I been so alive to the phenomenon of body, body as dwelling for life, as vessel for being, as vehicle for passage, as expression of the possibility of giving life to another human being. I have never been more present, more available to the astonishing presence of my own life, more aware of the wonder of the vessel "body."

Systems of human care must address and be a match for the magnificence of the human being incorporation. Traditional acupuncture is one of these systems—a powerful life medicine, a system of caring, of attending and giving utterance to our corporeal lives as stewards for life itself.

Pain is a powerful call to enter anew places that I thought I knew. When I "have" a headache, it is as though I have walked through a gate into a field called headache. I am lost. The headache has me. I belong to it, and I see no way to find myself. I must go through it. I must enter this familiar head into an unfamiliar experience, an experience that I interpret and fight as bad. The head I thought I knew, I have now opened some new questions about, and though I do not like my head with an ache, it does prompt me to see my head as a phenomenon about which I do not know everything. It may even be a moment for profound insight about being home. The French phenomenologist, Gabriel Marcel, spoke of participation rather than mere spectatorship as a fundamental of human existence. To him, sensation is the most elementary form of participation in being, rather than a mere receiving of messages from outside. It may be that our pains are our biggest way home, our most urgent call to Being. Perhaps nothing else other than what we call pain would capture our attention so insistently and thoroughly. It may be that we have to be awakened to our nobility by some sort of wake-up call, and often that call is a sensation of pain in our body and psyche. The great stories of quests and journeys and pilgrimages throughout history underscore the way home as the capacity to transform a pain, a terrible circumstance, a frightful obstacle into an instrument for journeying home in the all-embracing journey of life. We forget. We need reminders, like a monastery bell that will stop us in midsentence and call us to life past our ordinary wakefulness and our already knowing-it-all. We need to listen. Pain summons us until we attend to the old familiar with a new wonder. Our lostness demands we find our way home.

"The fact is," said Rabbit, "we've missed our way somehow."

They were having a rest in a small sand-pit on the top of the Forest. Pooh was getting rather tired of that sand-pit, and suspected it of following them about, because whichever direction they started in, they always ended up at it, and each time, as it came through the mist at them, Rabbit said triumphantly, "Now I know where we are!" and Pooh said sadly, "So do I," and Piglet said nothing. He had tried to think of something to say, but the only thing he could think of was "Help, help!" and it seemed silly to say that, when he had Pooh and Rabbit with him.

"Well," said Rabbit, after a long silence in which nobody thanked him for the nice walk they were having, "we'd better get on, I suppose. Which way shall we try?"

"How would it be, "said Pooh slowly, "if, as soon as we're out of sight of this Pit, we try to find it again?"

"What's the good of that?" said Rabbit.

"Well," said Pooh, "we keep looking for Home and not finding it, so I thought that if we looked for this Pit, we'd be sure not to find it, which would be a Good Thing, because then we might find something that we *weren't* looking for, which might be just what we *were* looking for, really."

"I don't see much sense in that," said Rabbit . . . .

"If I walked away from this Pit, and then walked back to it, of *course* I should find it."

"Well, I thought perhaps you wouldn't," said Pooh. "I just thought."

"Try," said Piglet suddenly. "We'll wait here for you."

Rabbit gave a laugh to show how silly Piglet was, and walked into the mist. After he had gone a hundred yards, he turned and walked back again . . . . and after Pooh and Piglet had waited twenty minutes for him, Pooh got up.

"I just thought," said Pooh. "Now then, Piglet, let's go home."

"But, Pooh," cried Piglet, all excited, "do you know the way?"

"No," said Pooh. "But there are twelve pots of honey in my cupboard, and they've been calling to me for hours. I couldn't hear them properly before, because Rabbit would talk, but if nobody says anything except those twelve pots, I think, Piglet, I shall know where they are calling from. Come on."

— A. A. Milne, *The House at Pooh Corner*

Our stories are many, as many as we are—although in *O Pioneers* Willa Cather tells us there are probably only two or three human themes and they keep being played out fiercely as though for the first time. At the heart of our matter, our stories give the interpretation of the journey of our lives. At the source of the journey we are home, before making the distinctions being-story-journey-home. It is from there that the wondrous caller to life, Teilhard de Chardin, speaks in his book, *The Heart of Matter:*

'You had need of me in order to grow; and I was waiting for you in order to be made holy.

'Always you have, without knowing it, desired me; and always I have been drawing you to me . . . .

'Are you coming?'

Lines carved on Thomas Wolfe's gravestone from his own work:

The last voyage—the longest, the best—
Look Homeward, Angel.*

Excerpt from a letter written by Buckminster Fuller to a ten-year-old:

The things to do are: the things that need doing, that you see need to be done, and that no one else seems to see need to be done. Then you will conceive your own way of doing that which needs to be done—that no one else has told you to do or how to do it. This will bring out the real you that often gets buried inside a character that has acquired a superficial array of behaviors induced or imposed by others on the individual.

Try making experiments of anything you conceive and are intensely interested in. Don't be disappointed if something doesn't work. That is what you want to know—the truth about everything—and then the truth about combinations of things. Some combinations have such logic and integrity that they can work coherently despite non-working elements embraced in their system.

Whenever you come to a word with which you are not familiar, find it in the dictionary and write a sentence which uses that new word. Words are tools—and once you have learned how to use a tool you will never forget it. Just looking for the meaning of the word is not enough. If your vocabulary is comprehensive, you can comprehend both fine and large patterns of experience.

*"Angel" in the Rilkean sense, Being.

You have what is most important in life—initiative. Because of it, you wrote to me. I am answering to the best of my capability. You will find the world responding to your earnest initiative.

———————

The universe is transformation, life is opinion...take away the opinion, and then there is taken away the complaint, "I have been harmed." Take away the complaint, "I have been harmed," and the harm is taken away.

— Marcus Aurelius

Pass then through this little space of time conformably to nature, and end thy journey in content, just as an olive falls off when it is ripe, blessing nature who produced it, and thanking the tree on which it grew.

— Marcus Aurelius

Excerpt from *The Velveteen Rabbit* by Margery Williams:

"What is *REAL*?" asked the Rabbit one day, when they were lying side by side near the nursery fender, before Nana came to tidy the room. "Does it mean having things that buzz inside you and a stick-out handle?"

"Real isn't how you are made," said the Skin Horse. "It's a thing that happens to you. When a child loves you for a long, long time, not just to play with, but *REALLY* loves you, then you become Real."

"Does it hurt?" asked the Rabbit.

"Sometimes," said the Skin Horse, for he was always truthful. "When you are Real you don't mind being hurt."

"Does it happen all at once, like being wound up," he asked, "or bit by bit?"

"It doesn't happen all at once," said the Skin Horse. "You become. It takes a long time. That's why it doesn't often happen to people who break easily, or have sharp edges, or who have to be carefully kept. Generally, by the time you are Real, most of your hair has been loved off, and your eyes drop out and you get loose in the joints and very shabby. But these things don't matter at all, because once you are Real you can't be ugly, except to people who don't understand."

Symptoms are ways home. They are our routes, our passages, our betaking of ourselves. A symptom is a kind of sigh, a sort of relief in a routine of life, a letting go of the familiar and entering of the unfamiliar. It is not a dangling part, but rather a striking, integrated expression of self. In the system of interpretation of traditional acupuncture, the symptom acts as a leitmotif, a main theme of a person's life that has been called up to be dealt with, to be completed. The symptom is not for the sake of itself. It is, rather, an instrument for wholing, healing, coming home.

The symptom sits in the person's history. It is a request for support; not support for simply getting rid of, or fixing it; but support for bearing it, for suffering it as an experience of life (*sub*, beneath + *ferre*, bear = suffering, undergoing); support for seeing the wisdom and embraceability of the symptom. It may even be said that a symptom, no matter how awesome or terrible, is life requesting to be embraced in all its manifestations. It is a deeply personal challenge for each of us to "marry" life totally and completely, for better or for worse, richer or poorer, in sickness and in health until death. This is not a partial commitment. It is an invitation to expand, to include the whole of life. A symptom is a way in to the whole, to the person's story, to her history, to her "storied" life. Like any opening, any way in, there are things that come into view right away, so, the symptom acts as an opening to vision and relationship beyond the ordinary, beyond the suffering.

We open our doors when we want someone to enter. We have doors because we anticipate that someone will enter. We give ourselves entrance. A door is also an exit, a way out, a place to move through toward someplace else. If I can show you something of myself, and a symptom is a "show," a showing, a manifestation, the most sanctioned-in-our-culture way to attend to ourselves, if I can take you to me through the door, and if you are willing to come with me, I will continue to lead us deeper into self. If you will come with me then into those places of myself, my life, my story where I have been alone, your very being with me enables me to come home to myself. When it is no longer needed as a touchstone, that is, as an entrance or exit, the symptom will disappear. It will reappear as it is needed. The theme of the life story will relax its grip on me and become a trustworthy companion presenting itself in new, strengthening and life-enhancing ways. Where I have been in such struggle a kind of power will emerge.

Let's use a specific symptom, a headache, to illustrate the preceding assertions. We could use any and all symptoms for this—insomnia, back pain, ulcers, depression, cancer, stress, etc.—and so I suggest that you, listener, substitute here whatever symptom you choose and see what opens up for you personally in this inquiry. The first thing I want to know is everything about the patient's experience of the headache (your headache). The label headache is insufficient. I ask her to inquire with me into her symptom and conduct an investigation so we can begin to make some opening in it. I ask her to tell me everything about it, tell me where her head hurts, what it feels like, what color it is, whether it is pain or ache, when does it come, when did she first experience it, what has she done to take care of it, what has she heard about headaches, do other family members have headaches, what are her fears about it, what has she seen and read about it, what does she remember going on in her life when she first had a headache, what is her ongoing conversation about it, what's her hunch about it being her head and not her knee or some other part hurting, how does it serve her, how does it hinder her, what would life be like without it, what would free up if she let go of it? So she describes herself to me via the symptom and all her associations and interpretations. As she takes me with her, she hears herself, often for the first time. She is making connections, seeing her own story, hearing her own accounting of how life is, completing her listenings, speaking her concerns, having empowering insights into the unity and continuity of her own life. She experiences herself whole and heard. (For the purposes of this illustration I have not included other parts of the examination that contribute to the experience of being whole and heard. In the entirety of the examination not one aspect of the person's life is a "ho-hum." The unity of her entire life is taken seriously and inquired into as a phenomenon of her being alive.)

She has shared herself with me, another whole and other-than-herself person, so that she is no longer alone where she once was so lonely. She has created a relationship with me and therefore knows her own loving nature through what she has created. The symptom that once loomed larger than herself, larger even than life, becomes manageable and even welcomed (not necessarily liked) as a possibility for knowing more about herself. (It is in this context that acupuncture treatment takes place, that is, the context of relationship and openings. Each treatment is a promise of a new possibility.) She has a symptom. The symptom does not have her. It has become a passageway to herself and to relationship. It has become a servant in the kingdom of human being.

There are lots of signals, manifestations that discomfit us, that we would not call symptoms ordinarily, yet really also warrant an inquiry. For example, a person wakes up in the morning and doesn't feel like getting out of bed. She experiences fatigue and calls it her "morning blahs," a label of her own making. She thinks of herself as a "night person," not a "morning person." And so, I ask her about herself via this symptom. Imagine, and it is not all that uncommon, having a part of the day, every day lost to you, especially the part that is the greeting of the day. The glory of the morning is lost for this person. She is not alive to herself, to a whole part of her life. As she describes her experience telling me her feelings, her reasons, her thoughts, dreams, hunches, memories, as she recreates the experience and takes me there with her, we look together into her life through this portal. This human being, like all of us human beings I dare say, wants to be present to her life, to miss none of it. It is that continual missing that all symptoms address. At the heart of us we want to be home, to be present to life, on the way home—moment by moment by moment by moment—forever.

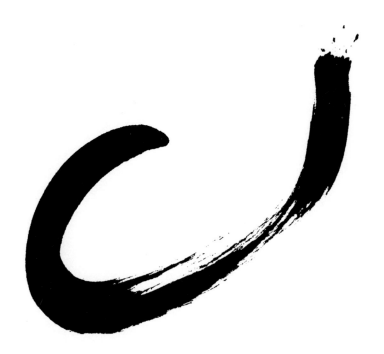

Shhh . . . . Inquire

CHAPTER SIX

Shhh . . . . Inquire

A child said *What is the grass?* fetching it to me
    with full hands,
How could I answer the child? I do not know what
    it is any more than he . . . .

               — Walt Whitman

. . . . the point is to live everything. Live the
questions now . . . .

               — Rainer Maria Rilke

Ask, and it shall be given you; seek, and you shall find;
knock, and it shall be opened to you.

               — Matthew 7:7

Hold every moment sacred. Give each clarity and
meaning, each the weight of thine awareness.

               — Thomas Mann

You could not find the end of the soul though you traveled everywhere, so deep is its logos.

— Heraclitus

To *inquire* is one of the four great diagnostic tools in Oriental medicine. To ask is to penetrate the mystery of one's being, to call forth. We gain entrance to each other by our questions, our callings to one another. In the question is a possibility. In the seeking for self is an opening for self. In the asking about symptom is an opening to the possibility within symptom, no matter what the symptom. In the inquiring into the familiar is an opening to the familiar. In the inquiry of who I am is a new possibility of who I am. In the search for home is a possibility of home. When I use the word "possibility" here I mean it as a new seeing, a looking beyond our old interpretations. By possibility I mean a new listening, or as ee cummings would say, "the ears of my ears awake."

My soul has lost its potentiality. If I were to wish for anything, I should not wish for wealth and power, but for the passionate sense of the potential, for the eye which, ever young and ardent, sees the possible . . . . what so fragrant, what so intoxicating, as possibility!

— Søren Kierkegaard

Did you ever think about the surprising texture of seeking? He who seeks does not have, he does not even know what he seeks, and on the other hand, to seek is to assume the thing sought and indeed to have it by prevision.

— Ortega y Gasset

We are coming from where we are going. "Seek ye the Kingdom? It is within." "Ask and it will be given you." The question "Who are you?" has "you" already at the heart of it. When I ask "you" who you are and you come with me into the quest, we are already in partnership, already home in our intention to navigate the question into both known and unknown territory of you, human being. I ask you and you give me yourself. I call to you and your life pours forth. I take you in, no matter what the content of your offerings, your sufferings, your expressions of humanity, of life as you know it, of life as it shows present and absent for you.

> With the drawing of this Love and the voice of
>   this Calling
> We shall not cease from exploration
> And the end of all our exploring
> Will be to arrive where we started
> And know the place for the first time.
> Through the unknown, remembered gate . . . .
>
> — T. S. Eliot

This is the nature of the diagnostic tool to inquire. The questions at the heart of another person's life, when voiced, create an opening, a possibility of life in the very asking. The inquiry is a plunge, a plummet, a plumb to the depths and surfaces of all life's data, all that we "know" currently and interpret as meaning one thing or another. In the question is a request to open beyond the old interpretations and look newly and not alone this time, but with the chosen partner, the practitioner, the inquiring one, the one committed to me being home in myself, the one willing to conduct the inquiry using herself as an instrument of my peace, of my possibility. In moving into and beyond our old stories about how life is, we require a practitioner-partner who is committed to mastering the art of inquiry, and mastering the art of the other diagnostic tools of listening, seeing, touching (feeling).

This is the enormous challenge and opportunity in being a practitioner (and here I would include that a practitioner of any endeavor is summoned to the same mastery that traditional acupuncture calls for, no matter what the discipline), the challenge of practicing, of putting into action the living of life as a daily inquiry, as an ongoing looking newly into the old. In the willingness of the practitioner to commit herself to mastery, the possibility of mastery arises for both practitioner and patient simultaneously and spontaneously in the treatment room, and, I daresay, in life. By mastery I mean a way of being a human being that generates aliveness and openings in everyone. By mastery I mean the phenomenon exhibited by any human being whose commitment to life can not be dissuaded by circumstances, like the player who in the last minute of the game, even when her team is losing plays her heart out to the end. She is no less thoroughly engaged then than when she is hitting a home run. She demonstrates a power of command over her personal considerations and circumstances.

This commitment to life, this masterful way of being is what I would also call a healing presence, that is, a person in whose presence being alive matters, a person in whose presence I come to open to who I am. The power of the relationship between practitioner and patient, that is, the relationship between partners, is inherent in the traditional acupuncture examination. The diagnostic tool of inquiry reveals so much more than questions asked to get good answers. The tool occasions an opening, a new putting together of old material from a person's life. It invites new authorship of an old script. The inquiry is not a technique. It is a way of being.

In fifteen years of being practitioner-partner in traditional acupuncture I have been entrusted with hearing and inquiring into the lifestory of many people. In the kaleidoscope of this great human company, I have seen how powerful questions give ground to an infinity of personal possibilities. In my ongoing experience of practice, I see increasing and astonishing evidence that the tool *to inquire* makes enormous openings for claiming life anew. It is like a home run in baseball. As soon as the ball comes and the person hits it, there is an impact that goes way beyond the moment of the hit: the ball goes out past the boundaries of the field and serves to bring the hitter home. It also brings home anyone else on base. A powerful inquiry is like a home run: it makes a connection that goes beyond "reasonable" limits and it brings home not just one person, but everyone else on the field. It returns us home.

Here's an example of a home run question posed in Oxford, England, to one of my first patients, a young American named Drew. Drew came for treatment because of symptoms diagnosed as asthma, side effects from drugs for the asthma, nightmares of being attacked, dread upon waking in the morning, and difficulty in relating to women. I walked into the treatment room and there Drew sat in a lotus position on the treatment table, naked. I was shocked. First of all, patients usually keep their underwear on, but it wasn't that so much, it was the way Drew was looking at me—what I interpreted as lustful, though he appeared rather like a flower child. In my training as a practitioner I was taught to see that human beings are always "saying" what is going on even if not with words, and I could see that Drew was in trouble in himself. Even so, as a brand new practitioner, I only had my willingness to serve, and not much experiential wherewithal. I couldn't even remember what I was supposed to do to begin the examination. And then, I did the only thing I could think of from what I could see, which I later saw as an act of trust in him and myself—I asked him the only question I could think of, which was: "Drew, when did your mother last hold you?" He burst into tears. It was an amazing moment. The question went right home, right to the heart of his suffering, to his ground, his life's conversation. It was like a dam bursting. We were both deeply moved. The question arrived as a home run and he brought us both home.

He began to speak about himself and his life as he had it storied, i.e. interpreted, and I continued to invite him to inquire past his history, through his symptoms, to the possibilities of his life. From there, from that "home run," from that opening, his whole life began to open up, not just to me and to himself, but to everyone else around him. With the support of treatment Drew stopped his asthma and decided to change his sleep habits by going to bed later and getting up later. He sleeps fine with no nightmares now and only some mornings dreads getting up. He is now happily married and has two little children. In the course of treatment we became good friends.

In a question, any question, there is always an unknown, an X. What is to be known by inquiring into the nature of X, the unknown, is the nature of it. Bernard Lonergan, a Jesuit and one of my mentors in undergraduate school, commented on this unknown in his book *Insight: A Study of Human Understanding:*

> Just as in algebra the unknown number is x, until one finds out what the number is, so too in empirical inquiry, the unknown to be reached by insight is named "the nature of . . . ." Once Galileo discovered his law, he knew that the nature of a free fall was a constant acceleration. But before he discovered the law, from the mere fact that he inquired, he knew that a free fall possessed a nature, though he did not know what that nature was.

For a practitioner, then, every inquiry presumes the question, What is the nature of . . . . ? And, every phenomenon comes into view as a phenomenon about which I can ask What is the nature of . . . . ?, no matter how mundane or lofty, how physical or non-physical, how familiar or unfamiliar, how manifest or hidden is the subject of the inquiry. We desire to know the nature of things, of everything, of every phenomenon—the nature of symptom, of daily events, of relationship with food, sleep, vision, digestion, bowels, urination, breathing, circulation, sexuality, all the arenas of life, the nature of the questioner from whence comes the questions, the nature of human being, the nature of life itself, and so we ask. Asking makes us voyagers. It gives us movement that takes us traveling beyond our known selves into unknown selves. We begin to see that there is a lot to make an inquiry about, maybe everything, including Who is the one asking? Who are we, and Who are we that we even ask? What opens as a result of our askings?

In *What Is Philosophy?*, Ortega y Gasset suggests to us that what opens with inquiry is ". . . . feeling oneself live, knowing oneself to be existing—where knowing implies no intellectual knowledge nor special wisdom, but is that surprising presence which one's own life has for everyone of us: without that kind of knowing, without that recognition of itself, the aching tooth would not hurt us." What opens with inquiry is the presence of one's own life. Life is close by, "made up of all the things that are nearest to each of us."

Your life now consists of reading my words. This, and all the daily acts and events, the "furnishings," all of them are a "matter of life." Being present to my own life brings the world with it. As I experience myself alive and present I begin to engage with the fabric of life, all the Dianne-in-the-worldness that I am wakeful to. I begin to see how much I live life in the conversation that "something is wrong and needs to be fixed"—me, them, it. I begin to look more deeply into the stuff of my own life. Inquiry that opens the experience of my experience of life begets further inquiry into the "whats" I am present to. The "whats" for me include my children, my body, food, sleep, teaching, my practice, writing, my relationships. I begin to hear beyond my ordinary hearing to what I have heretofore perfunctorily called "life."

> Life is not a mystery, but quite the opposite; it is the clearest and most present thing there is, and being so, being purely transparent, we find difficulty in studying it closely.
>
> — Ortega y Gasset

The above statements about our life, and being present to one's life are the territory of this chapter, "Shhh . . . . Inquire." It is the territory of traditional acupuncture and, I assert, the territory of every human medicine with integrity. Being present to one's life is being home. It is the territory of the quest. All medicine concerns itself with the tools, resources, instruments that we need to navigate our way home, to guide us in the home stretch, to support us in diving deep into the day of our lives, the story of the me and you, the unexplored, incomplete, unexperienced experience of our lives. All healing is a homecoming, being present to my own life exactly as I am. I come as I am. My arrival is my life. Being present is the healing, no matter what the description of the "whats." As practitioner I am privileged to be here for the arrival of my partners, my patients, in their homecoming. This is the intimacy of the healing relationship. This is the possibility of a global homecoming. This is the joy in life, the power of inquiry, the wonder in being alive.

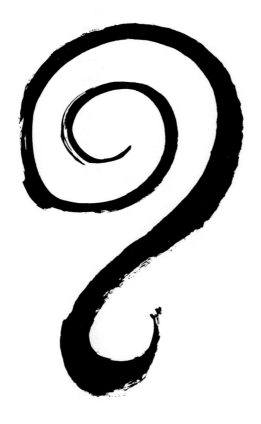

Shhh . . . . Listen

CHAPTER SEVEN

Shhh . . . . Listen

. . . . the pause . . . . a space yet unfilled . . . . a "no thing" . . . . is especially important for the freedom of being . . . . (it) gives us a whole new world. It is in the pause that people learn to *listen to silence.*

— Rollo May

If the unheard, unspoken
Word is unspoken, unheard;
Still is the unspoken word, the Word unheard,
The Word without a word, the Word within
The world and for the world;
And the light shone in darkness and
Against the Word the unstilled world still whirled
About the centre of the silent Word.
. . . .
Where shall the word be found, where will the word
Resound? Not here, there is not enough silence . . . .

— T. S. Eliot

Cease listening with the mind and listen with the
vital spirit . . . .

— Chuang Tze

. . . . the Word, coming forth from Silence,
leads . . . . home into Silence.

                                — Brother David Steindl-Rast

Only the twilight now, and the soft "Sh!" of the river
    That will last for ever.

                                — D. H. Lawrence

being to timelessness as it's to time, ...
love is the voice under all silences, ...

                                — ee cummings

I s there anything that we do not have a name and a
meaning for? We, human beings, name things and give
meanings to everything. If I say anything, any word or a
phrase, you are likely to have an association with it, a story
for it, an interpretation of it, an opinion about it, an already
knowing. Everything means something to us even if our
meanings about the same things differ; you and I are very
unlikely to listen a word, any word, brand new, putting it no
place, doing with it nothing. We will seek to find a history for
it, to remember the context we last heard it in. We will even
get upset if we have no memory or understanding of what is
said, as though we should "know."

    We ordinarily listen what we already know, and put things
into meanings that we made up long ago, either in our
personal or in our cultural history. Rarely do we not give our
experience a ready-made name and meaning; rarely do we
simply experience the wonder of human beings speaking,
human beings giving expression to their experience of life,
human beings making meanings, human beings making
words flesh.

    Two rather powerful and moving illustrations of what I'm
saying, illustrations of the wonder of language, of naming, of

being present to the moment of meaning's birth, come to mind. The first is the experience referred to often in almost any conversation regarding language, and that is the experience described by Helen Keller in her leaving of the silent wordless world in which she lived: "Someone was drawing water . . . . As the cool stream gushed over my hand she spelled into the other the word 'water' . . . . I stood still, my whole attention fixed upon the motion of her fingers. Suddenly I felt a misty consciousness as of something forgotten — a thrill of returning thought; and somehow the mystery of language was revealed to me."

The second illustration is the story of our first word, the word that heralds our verbal entrance into the family as a communicator. The baby says "dog" one day when the furry, moving creature comes into the room for the hundredth time. It is a day of great joy and celebration. A little human being has spoken a word, has given meaning to something, has become herself by distinguishing something outside herself and communicated it—in this instance "dog." Then comes the day when a furry, moving creature enters the room and baby says "dog" and mommy says "no, not dog, cat." And we begin to make distinctions among furry, moving things, naming as we go and remembering what makes what what. We make meaning and use words to represent our experience of "the world," so that if I say "dog" to you, without actually having the furry, moving creature present, you will think "dog" too. By my speaking a word I bring a world into existence between us—in this instance the world "dog." In the world "dog" there are hundreds of distinctions, lots of names, variations, descriptions, i.e., different expressions of "dogness," so one of the tasks of a human being is to learn to speak distinctions, that is, to speak and in speaking create the world. Heidegger asserted that human beings dwell in the house of language and that language is the "house of being." We speak to each other and in so doing we bring forth the world for each other. So, it matters what words we use and what our listening is, that is, what worlds we call forth. In words we carry the world with us.

A distinguished philosopher of language, Fernando Flores, asserts that listening grants speaking, and that speaking is close to who we are. Listening grants speaking. Take this in. If you give me your listening, I have a place for my speaking, a partner in bringing forth a world with my words, and so my words become more than vibrations of the air and sound waves, they become worlds, conversations between human beings creating what Martin Buber called "I-Thou," and ee cummings called "little you-i." T. S. Eliot said,". . . . where every word is at home, taking its place to support the others." I pour myself into your listening. I give you my words, my worlds, my life. You home me. You, through your listening, give me dwelling. You give me residence. You, being, grant me, being.

What are we listening? In, through, between, among the words, what are we attending? To what do I harken and give back to you in my speaking into your listening? What is the dialogue of creation? To what am I listening? When the monastery bell sounds its call to silence, where must I go to respond to the call? Am I not summoned to listen creation, to attend being, to be present to self? Is "home" in my listening? Is that not the greatest of human gifts? Give me your listening and together we bring forth the world. I give you my listening, and you speak your life. Together we create home, our life, our homecoming to being.

Herein we enter the land of paradox, the land beyond reason, the land from which we build toward the unknown:

> Tao is the Tao that can not be spoken . . . .
> Listen to it, but you can not hear it!
> Its name is "Soundless."
>
> — Lao Tze

Not known, because not looked for
But heard, half-heard, in the stillness
Between two waves of the sea.
Quick now, here, now, always—
A condition of complete simplicity
(Costing not less than everything)

— T. S. Eliot

Perhaps we can not say the Truth, but, we can "true" up, that is, we can bring creation home to itself, to its own authentic knowing. In Chinatown in San Francisco there is a bridge along which are tableaus depicting the virtues. One of the virtues is called "The Four Knows"; the tableau depicts the story of one man attempting to bribe another, saying ". . . . and, no one knows," to which the other says "Whatever do you mean, no one knows? There are four who know: Heaven knows, Earth knows, You know and I know."

And although we can not speak the Tao, what we can do is promise our humanity as godly, thereby including the entirety of our human life as creative and recreat-able. Perhaps I can listen you as Self, listen you as the unity of your selves. Perhaps we can stand together at "the still point of the turning world" and listen intently the word of Silence from which all speaking comes, listen intently the Word of words for which all listening is meant, listen the Tao which can not be heard.

It is wise to listen, ... not to me but to the Word, and to confess that all things are one . . . .

— Heraclitus

It is in the cradle of this conversation about language that I have written "Shhh . . . . Listen." One of the four great diagnostic tools of Oriental medicine is *To Listen*. It requires "a condition of complete simplicity." It requires a stillness, an emptiness, a silence, a "shhh," an unknowing. It requires us to hearken the soundless, the silence before, during, after the words. By diagnostic tool I mean an instrument by which to diagnose,* that is, by which to make distinctions to determine the nature of something, and to act according to that nature. To listen my patients, is to listen the "what" of their lives: yet, even more powerfully, listening is the instrument that allows "that" they are alive to show. The diagnostic instrument of listening creates an opening not simply to eliminate symptoms, but also to create life as an opening.

> All that we do
> Is touched with ocean, yet we remain
> On the shore of what we know.
>
> — Richard Purdy Wilbur

My work in the treatment room is to be still, to be home in myself, and into my stillness comes a request from my patient to listen her, to "unknow" her, that is, to listen her "already knowings" of herself as she gives me her words and her worlds of meanings, the stories and interpretations that she has already created to live her life by. She summons me to listen her new, as unknown, as possibility. To hear the sounds of health and sickness, I can not already know her. I must stand in the silence of not knowing, listening, no matter what she is saying, the unknown, the worlds not yet named, and the meanings not yet given, the paradox that truth is unspeakable even as we listen to the speaking.

> Now I will do nothing but listen,
> To accrue what I hear into this song . . . .
>
> — Walt Whitman

---

*"Diagnosis" usually refers to illness, disease, sickness. Other words associated with diagnosing are examining, investigating, probing, looking into, distinguishing, characterizing.

All waits for the right voices;
Where is the practis'd and perfect organ? Where is the
    develop'd soul?
For I see every word utter'd thence has deeper,
    sweeter, new sounds,
        impossible on less terms.

I see brains and lips closed, tympans and temples
    unstruck,
Until that comes which has the quality to strike and to
    unclose,
Until that comes which has the quality to bring forth
    what lies
        slumbering forever ready in all words.

                    — Walt Whitman

Voices. Voices. Listen, my heart, as only
saints have listened: until the gigantic call lifted them
off the ground; yet they kept on, impossibly,
kneeling and didn't notice at all:
so complete was their listening. Not that you could
    endure
God's voice—far from it. But listen to the voice of the
    wind
and the ceaseless message that forms itself out of
silence.

                    — Rainer Maria Rilke

Creatures of stillness . . . . quiet in themselves,
. . . . from simply listening . . . .

. . . . you built a temple deep inside their hearing.

                    — Rainer Maria Rilke

May my silences become more accurate.

                    — Theodore Roethke

Tom came to me, a man in his mid-fifties, suffering what he called the "wounds and arrows" of life. His wife of thirty years had left him. He had pains in his chest—"my heart pangs." A project associated with his position as professor in a university was overdue. He was overwhelmed and could not function enough to cook a meal for himself. He said, "I am forlorn and lost. All the things I held dear are falling apart. Life looks impossible from here." Now, as a practitioner, hearing all this, I wanted to take it from him, just wipe the slate of his life clean and give him a brand new start. I could not give him that, but what I could give him was my listening. My listening had no boundaries for how Tom could heal himself, and so, quite like James Joyce and the "stream of consciousness" Tom spoke into the listening. He gave me his life. I held his life and embraced and continued to hold this human life pouring forth; his words were his life blood, and I the container for receiving the precious fluid. Through it all I could hear the sounds of life, of his suffering, of the things he liked and the things he despised, the cadence and music of one human life. "And, what else, Tom . . . . what else . . . . what else . . . . yes, that too, and what else," all the while observing my own desire to jump in and add to or take away from his life as presented. I danced in my listening, alternating between being an empty vessel, a clearing, in which his life would appear, and desiring to change this expression of life. Except for the "and, what else" I remained silent for his speaking. As a practitioner I do not always stay silent, yet for Tom I thought perhaps in the silence he would find an opening in the knot of his life, even before we had any treatment with needles. His life appeared like a knot so tight and constricting to him that he could not see anything beyond the circumstances. For Tom his personal life was nowhere in sight of life as gift or possibility. And so, I listened life as he spoke his life. Finally, not yet at the end of the examination, he put his forefinger to his mouth as if to hush a child, and he said "Shhh, Dianne, listen." He had his eyes closed with tears streaming down his face as though he was listening to something enormously moving to him. "I hear my own life," he said. And what I heard was the awesome arrival of life coming home to itself.

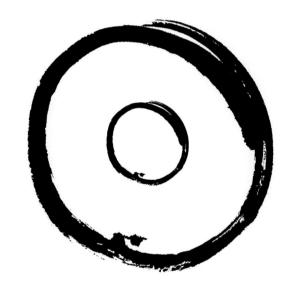

Seeing

CHAPTER EIGHT

Seeing

(Dedicated to my mother)

Now the eyes of my eyes are opened . . . .

— ee cummings

While going down a slope, Zorba kicked against a stone, which went rolling downhill. He stopped for a moment in amazement, as if he were seeing this astounding spectacle for the first time in his life. He looked round at me, and in his look I discerned faint consternation.

"Boss, did you see that?" he said at last. "On slopes, stones come to life again."

I said nothing, but I felt a deep joy. This, I thought, is how great visionaries and poets see everything—as if for the first time. Each morning they see a new world before their eyes; they do not really see it, they create it.

The universe for Zorba, as for the first men on earth, was a weighty, intense vision; the stars glided over him, the sea broke against his temples. He lived the earth, water, the animals and God, without the distorting intervention of reason.

— Nikos Kazantzakis

Give me the looks that recall me.

— James Dickey

. . . . and then
I could not see to see.

— Emily Dickinson

This chapter is for you, Mom. It is about vision, about seeing. One day, in my first acupuncture class, my professor, Dr. Worsley, said to us, "You think you see, but you don't. The day you really see you will weep. You will be moved to tears at the magnificence of a tree, the petals of a flower, the hands of an infant. And then, then you begin to open your eyes to everything, to everyone, and really see beyond what you have seen before." As he spoke I thought of you, Mama, in all your shyness about your unseeing eye, you have given me seeing, you have given me to wonder, to stand in awe at the gift of sight.

To see is one of the four basic tools of diagnosis in traditional acupuncture. The power and the simplicity of seeing is not just in what we see and what we have room to see, but also in that we see. In entering a life's work in which the instrument of vision is so central to it, in fact, at the heart of it, I am always coming home, home from where I started, and home where I am heading. I see. God, what a statement! It is no wonder that in conversation when we understand something or experience a connection, what we say is I see, I see what you mean, I see what you are saying, I see you, I see. It is both a beginning and an ending, or perhaps more aptly said, a moment of no beginning and no end. Perhaps all visionaries, like Mother Theresa, for example, have one eye on the oozing sores and the hungry to be fed, and one eye on the godliness of humanity. Perhaps a visionary is one who lives her life in "I see," in a vision large enough to hold all of

90

the conditions of life—never losing sight of the heart of all matter.

Life's challenge, first posed to me by my mother, is the seeing—or as in Zorba—the creating of a new world, a world anew. My mother sees—creates the flower in everything. She looks with "the eyes of her eyes." She takes what someone else might call a lifetime handicap—she has only one eye—and makes of it a triumphant gift of sight, an exaltation of human possibility, a new vision. My mother's lifelong coaching taught me not to miss the requests from my patients to look with them at their life, their symptom, their story as an asking for new sight, for an opening, a seeing beyond their present looking.

What we see guides us. My children teach me seeing, too. Three years ago, just before Halloween, I was in England supervising an American acupuncture class. Since I'd be arriving in the United States on Halloween afternoon, I called home to talk to my children about their plans. My girl child, Jade, answered with great excitement: "Mommy, I'm going to be a Rubik's cube for Halloween. I made the costume myself and I'm going to wear it to the airport when we come to pick you up." Then, she faltered, hesitated, and continued very seriously, "So, Mommy, when you see a little kid dressed like a Rubik's cube, be sure and come up and say, Little kid, little kid, are you Jade?' "

Through her words, I could see all of us, all of us human kids, saying to each other, "Don't miss me, no matter what costume I'm in." And, we do mean it with grave seriousness. We have excitement and pride in our costumes, our get-ups, our visible creations, our credentials, our accoutrements, and yet within all of it, within each of our Rubik's cubes, we of the who-we-really-are want not to be missed.

There is a story attributed to Lieh Tzu about the Duke of Mu and of his legendary advisor on horses, Po Lo (Uncle Happy). The Duke said to Po Lo one day, "You are getting very old. Is there anyone in your family who could find me a horse?" Po Lo replied, "To find a good horse, you must look at its shape, conformation, muscle and bone: but to find a Heavenly Horse, you must forget all these things. My sons are of the lesser talent: they could find you a good horse, but not a Heavenly Horse. There's an old man I know, who is a carrier of vegetables and firewood: he knows as much about horses as I ever did; please see him."

The Duke saw this old man, who went away and after three months returned saying "I've found it!" The Duke said: "What sort of horse is it?" and the old man replied "A dun mare." The Duke asked for it to be led in. The horse was a stallion and black. The Duke was not pleased and called for Po Lo. To Po Lo he said, "This man you sent me can't even tell the color or sex of a horse! How could you say he was a man who knew all about horses?"

Po Lo sighed deeply and said, "Oh, is he as good as that now? It is as if, when he looks at a horse, there are more important things to him than horses!"

This story is a demonstration of how what we see guides us. Do I have room for a Heavenly Horse to show up past my pictures of what I already know called horse? Where am I looking to find you? What is the act of seeing? "I wish I could find an event that meant as much as simple seeing!" (Theodore Roethke) We are always starting with what we see. What is the biggest vision I can have of you? How do I find a Heavenly person? My seeing is sufficient only when it includes all of all of you.

> I love in-seeing. Can you imagine with me how glorious it is to in-see a dog, for example, as you pass it—by in-see I don't mean to look through, which is only a kind of human gymnastic that lets you immediately come out again on the other side of the dog, regarding it merely, so to speak, as a window upon the human world lying behind it: not that; what I mean is to let yourself precisely into the dog's center, the point from which it begins to be a dog, the place in it where God, as it were, would have sat down for a moment when the dog was finished, in order to watch its first embarrassments and inspi-

rations and to nod that it was good, that nothing was lacking, that it couldn't have been better made. . . . my world-feeling, my earthly bliss was . . . . in such in-seeing—in the indescribably swift, deep, timeless moments of this godlike in-seeing.

— Rainer Maria Rilke

Healing is seeing. Healers are visionaries willing and determined to see unity and peace. We are all healers. It is time to open our eyes, to see who we are, to have a vision big enough to include all of each of us and every facet of ourselves. We are here together and we are here for life. As individuals and as world people we count on each other to have sight . . . . to know who we really are at the very core of our being . . . . to provide vision for one another when we are blind to ourselves . . . . to create life as a partnership. For brief moments we are in danger of being fooled by appearances . . . . in danger of taking the layers of life's accumulations, the chapters of our story, the rhythms of our daily hum as though they are not a chosen part of our healing. We reach for the symptoms as problems to be discarded rather than opportunities to realize the integrity of our bodymindspirit. Every moment of life, be it in intimacy or in politics, requires us to acknowledge and reveal our Nature. By the very force of life, we are commanded to know who we are so that we see every interchange as a source of nourishment, every moment as making a difference, every relationship as a source of empowerment, every symptom as a sign of integrity. Herein lies the healing, the coming into wholeness, the making room for each other in the recognition of our deep and ineluctable journey . . . . creating vision and furthering life. In this we find our purpose . . . . into this the light comes piercing . . . . from this we see anew.

> While with an eye made quiet by the power
> Of harmony, and the deep power of joy,
> We see into the life of things

— William Wordsworth

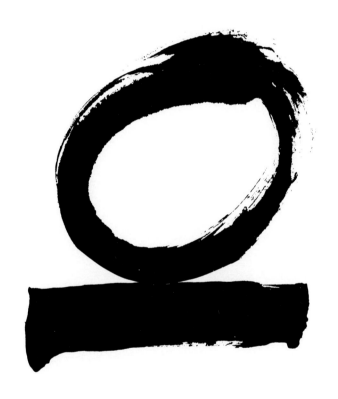

I Give You My Hand

CHAPTER NINE

I Give You My Hand

Camerado, I give you my hand!
I give you my love more precious than money,
I give you myself before preaching or law;
Will you give me yourself? will you come travel
    with me?
Shall we stick by each other as long as we live?

— Walt Whitman

"Saint Francis and the Sow"

The bud
stands for all things,
even for those things that don't flower,
for everything flowers from within, of self-blessing;
though sometimes it is necessary
to reteach a thing its loveliness,
to put a hand on its brow
of the flower
and retell it in words and in touch
it is lovely
until it flowers again from within, of self-blessing;
as Saint Francis

put his hand on the creased forehead
of the sow, and told her in words and in touch
blessings of earth on the sow, and the sow
began remembering all down her thick length,
from the earthen snout all the way
through the fodder and slops to the spiritual curl
    of the tail,
from the hard spininess spiked out from the spine
down through the great broken heart
to the blue milken dreaminess spurting and shuddering
from the fourteen teats into the fourteen mouths
    sucking and
blowing beneath them:
the long, perfect loveliness of sow.

— Galway Kinnell

The human body is the magazine of inventions, the patent office, where are all the models from which every hint is taken. All the tools and engines in earth are only extensions of its limbs and senses.

— Ralph Waldo Emerson

T o *feel* is one of the four main diagnostic tools in Oriental medicine. What is it to feel? The dictionaries state that *to feel* is to perceive, as by the *touch*; to examine by touching, to be mentally affected or stirred by, to be conscious of, to have a sense of, to have a sensation of being, to be moved, to have a specific sensation by touch, to consider oneself to be; to be conscious of being, to find one's way by touch . . . .

I work with my hands. It is a great privilege to touch another human being, to remind her in word and in touch that she is lovely, to put a hand on the brow of life and call her home. The wonder of touch is the wonder of human kindness. Never is the needle more than an extension of person touching person. A giving of one's hand is a giving of

one's life, one's word, one's promise, one's blessing. It is a gift
of the highest order, as forgiveness and compassion. "You
can do nothing and be nothing but what I will infold you."
(Walt Whitman)

Hands, hands that hold babies, that take pulses, that insert
needles, that hold hands; hands that touch life; my hands,
your hands, human hands. Richard Seltzer in *Mortal Lessons*
describes the Dalai Lama's physician taking the pulses of a
patient:

> . . . . their hands are joined in a correspondence that is
> exclusive, intimate, his fingertips receiving the voice of her
> sick body through the rhythm and throb she offers at her
> wrist. All at once I am envious—not of him, not of Yeshi
> Dhonden for his gift of beauty and holiness, but of her. I want
> to be held like that, touched so, "received."

Touching prompts a recollection of being, a "remem-
brance of things past," a recurring to oneself through the
body. With my hands on her scarred knees during the examination, my patient Elizabeth blurted out that she was afraid,
that the pain in her knees was excruciating. She kept talking
and revealing how terrified she was when at six years of age,
she ran to tell someone her baby brother had fallen into the
pond near their house. She had fallen and skinned her knees
then, and subsequently had fallen many times during her
childhood and into her adult years. One of her reasons for
coming for treatment was the physical pain in her knees and
hips, as well as an impending sense of doom about her life.

Stephen, another patient, came for treatment originally
because of ear problems he had had all his life—lots of
earaches, ear infections, hearing loss. He began to cry as I
ever so gently touched his ears. He told me about his wonderful old grandfather who lived with him as a child, and who
would hold him and sing to him when he had an earache—
sing softly and cooingly some old Irish songs. His grandfather had died abruptly, all very secretive when Stephen

was ten years old, and no one ever talked to Stephen about what happened. He reported: "I feel that I am still listening for my grandfather, waiting for him to hold me again." Stephen is fifty years old.

Gandhi said, "Work with the hands is the apprenticeship of honesty. May the work of your hands be a sign of gratitude and reverence to the human condition." Through our hands we touch that which comes out of the universe, that which is the vessel of life, matter itself, the abode, the body. The corporate, collective, functioning "body" is known to us through touch and feel, through examination and exploration. It is an infinite kingdom to explore and open to. We describe ourselves through our bodies. We have our residence in the body for the space and time we call life, our lifetime, our lifespace. All we have is life to live and our transporting vessel for aliveness is body. Little do I know the extent of my identity with my body until I am touched. Little am I present to body, my body, until a hand is laid upon me calling me to the "temple," to the housing of my self, to the homing of my spirit, to the dwelling of my existence. The wonder of a physical symptom is the call that it is in my body, a call to be touched, to attend my pain through my body, the vessel that houses me. My body's predicament always points beyond itself. The hand that touches my body touches my life. My body is in me. I sing with it, talk with it, fatten it, skinny it, eat with it, sleep with it. I do everything including "be" in my body. So, when you touch me, the "commons" of me, my body, you enter my life, my being, you come into my dwelling—no matter where you touch me. Touch always involves the presence of the body, my own and the other's. Touch presences. I am touched by you, moved by your presence.

> . . . . I recall a hand resting on another person, in which there is concentrated a contact that remains infinitely remote from any touch, something that may not even be called gesture any

longer in the sense in which I understand your usage. For this
hand is suffused and borne by a call calling from afar and
calling still farther onward, because stillness has brought it.

— Martin Heidegger

To give life, but to claim nothing.

— Lao Tze

To see a World in a Grain of Sand
And a Heaven in a Wild flower,
Hold Infinity in the palm of your hand,
And Eternity in an hour.

— William Blake

. . . . and if ever i touched a life i hope that life
    knows
that i know that touching was and still is and
    always will be the true
revolution

— Nikki Giovanni

now here was I, new-awakened, with my hand stretching out
and touching the unknown, the real unknown, the unknown
unknown.

— D. H. Lawrence

It is not possible that we have nothing to contribute to one
another. Whatever anyone has given me, that you can have
from me. Others have given me their touch, their tenderness,
their acknowledgment of my life. I give you my touch, my
acknowledgment of your body, of your life.

Touch me, touch the palm of your hand to my body as I pass,
Be not afraid of my body.

— Walt Whitman

I wish to infuse myself among you till I see it common for you
to walk hand in hand.

— Walt Whitman

To touch my person to someone else's is about as much as I
can stand.

— Walt Whitman

All truths wait in all things . . . .
(What is less or more than a touch?)

— Walt Whitman

Since this is the last night I keep you home.
Come, I will consecrate you for the journey.

— D. H. Lawrence

All of the preceding quotes, words on touching, on giving
ourselves, our hands to each other, are a perfect setting for
one of the main uses of our hands as an acupuncture practitioner, and that is the taking of the pulses. We are instructed
by the classics that where blood flows, the Ch'i, the force of
life itself, flows. To find a major artery, a place where the
blood flows, and then, locate there the Ch'i and feel the flow
of life itself, that is known as taking the pulses. It requires
what Heidegger referred to as a hand "suffused and borne
by a call," having been brought to its place by "stillness."
There are twelve readings of the Ch'i to locate, each corres-
ponding to an "orb," "official," "charge." (See the Postscript
on the Three-Heater.) Holding another's hand with my hand
to take her pulses, to "read" her life force, is of great
moment. With eyes closed, silence in the room, and fingers
over the radial arterial blood pulse, I attend. So does my
patient. We listen together, present to the life of her life. My
hands are the bodily bridge between us, as later the needle
will be when it enters the point of choice to give witness, to
create connection, to clear the way.

Jacques Lusseyran, blind from the age of eight, wrote of touching:

> Touching the tomatoes in the garden, and really touching them, touching the walls of the house, the materials of the curtains or a clod of earth is surely seeing them as fully as eyes can see. But it is more than seeing them, it is tuning in on them and allowing the current they hold to connect with one's own, like electricity. To put it differently, this means an end of living in front of things and a beginning of living with them. Never mind if the word sounds shocking, for this is love.
>
> You cannot keep your hands from loving what they have really felt . . . .

"Camerado, I give you my hand!" Our work is to bear each other home, to take care of each other. I personally can think of nothing more wonderful than to be the handmaiden of life, to serve as an instrument of peace on my way home, no matter how many times in a day I may forget to reach out my hand. This work reminds me of my stewardship. In concluding this chapter I give you one of my favorite passages, which speaks of this chapter's theme:

> Lord, make me an instrument of your peace.
> Where there is hatred let me sow love.
> Where there is injury—pardon.
> Where there is doubt—faith.
> Where there is despair—hope.
> Where there is darkness—light.
> Where there is sadness—joy.
>
> O Divine Master, grant that I may not so much seek
> To be consoled as to console
> To be understood as to understand
> To be loved as to love.
> For, it is in giving that we receive.
> It is in pardoning that we are pardoned.
> It is in dying that we are born to eternal life.
>
> — Prayer of St. Francis of Assisi

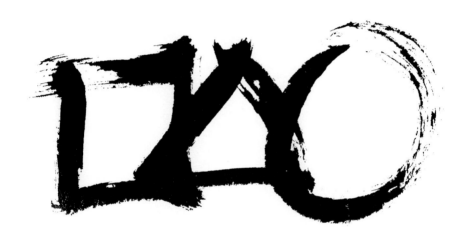

Great Oneness

CHAPTER TEN

Great Oneness*

(To the students)

When the ten thousand things are viewed in their oneness, we return to the origin and remain where we have always been.

— Lao Tze

You don't live in a world all alone. Your brothers are here too.

— Albert Schweitzer

Rain is no respecter of persons
the snow doesn't give a soft white
damn Whom it touches

— ee cummings

*"Great Oneness" is a translation of the Chinese characters for the acupuncture point known as Stomach 23.

> the sky covers
> the earth carries
> and the sun and moon shine upon,
> no one in particular
>
> — San Wu

The rainstorm is not personal, and yet we get personally wet.

— Werner Erhard

> love is a place
> & through this place of
> love move
> (with brightness of peace)
> all places
>
> yes is a world
> & in this world of
> yes live
> (skilfully curled)
> all worlds
>
> — ee cummings

T he theme of this chapter is spoken in the above quotes. Life is a nonpersonal force, and yet we are personally alive. I am not personal to the snow, to the rain, to the sky, the earth, the sun and moon, to nature, and yet my experience of them and relationship to them is profoundly personal, intimate to me. The sun shines on each of us equally. One single sun illuminates the whole human family. It doesn't care who I am, who you are. None of our personal detail matters. Our personal wetness, our personal warmth, our personalness is held in the great impersonal life force making of us brothers and sisters, giving to us the underlying common union, returning us to our origin, balancing all unequal appearances, homing our "no-one, anyone, someone, everyone" self. (ee cummings) The seasons come and go whether we want them to or not. The life cycle continues before us and after us generation after generation. Nature mates life with life through wilderness and clearings, storms and calms, season through season, day by day, hour by hour. Life itself holds the lifes of us. In life all lifes. Before our own personal births and after our personal deaths, life.

> And, who art thou? said I to the soft-falling shower,
> . . . .
> I am the Poem of Earth, said the voice of the rain,
> Eternal I rise impalpable out of the land and the bottomless
>   sea
>   . . . .
> And forever, by day and night, I give back life to my own
>   origin and make pure and beautify it . . . .
>
>   — Walt Whitman

The pathways of the life force, and the points along the paths are inclusive of everyone. All of humanity regardless of name, age, color, sex, culture, occupation, location, size, shape, standards, beliefs—all participate in the vastly reaching interpretations of the life force, the impersonal Ch'i, in a personal claiming. The points belong to all of us equally. Life "lives" each of us and every acupuncture point, every meridian pathway calls us to that life. "Listening Palace," "Great Esteem," "Gate of Life," "Inner Courtyard," "Great Oneness," "Abundant Splendor," "People Welcome," "Heavenly Pivot," "Great Enveloping": every single acupuncture point is a call to each of us, all of the time, equally, equitably. The life force is nonpersonal, that is to say, indifferent to the individual that we say we are. We personalize life in the living of our life. Each point is impersonal. We personalize them in the use of them, in the naming of them. Points become entrances into our lives. They move us to unravel what we have taken to be very personal, what we have created as our own personalities out of the myriad possibilities in the nonpersonal universe. Each point supports us in some aspect of our person, some letting go of old baggage, cleaning up of messes, removing of barriers, clarifying of where we have collapsed the distinctions of impersonal with personal, that is, where we have taken life events as a personal affront when it has simply been life like a rainstorm, not designed to get me personally wet.

This conversation reminds me of the story of the fellow who looks up in the sky, and a bird flying overhead poops on his shoulder; he sighs and says: "For other people they sing!" We continually interpret life as being for or against us. We even take the weather personally. On a day off it rains; when I'm working it's sunny, as though nature really is out to "get" me. And, we interpret each other very personally, as though someone else's individual storm is designed for us personally. If someone, especially someone close to me is "storming," it is difficult to allow them their weather without taking it personally and getting very wet. It may be that our individual weather is never personal except as we make it so. It may be that we are always taking life personally, seeing ourselves as our titles and our personal particulars. Perhaps the source of struggle and suffering comes from identifying life with any particular life, rather than all life as manifest through each of us.

> Without the transcendent and the transpersonal, we get sick .
> . . . or else hopeless and apathetic. We need something "bigger than we are" to be awed by and to commit ourselves to . . . .
>
> — Abraham Maslow

What Maslow called the transcendent and the transpersonal, I am calling the impersonal, or nonpersonal. It may be that all of our human conditions and expressions of that humanity are manifestations of nature, of the life force ever unfolding through us, ultimately encompassing all the varia-

tion of life, known only through actually living and personalizing the ebbs and flows, the nights and days, the comings
and goings, leavings and returnings, alivenesses and dead-
nesses, holding on and letting go, littles and bigs, noises and
quiets, birthings and dyings, all the ten thousand, the infinite,
the nonpersonal, the myriad things.

Pere Claude Larre, S.J., a French Jesuit sinologist, translates the Chinese classics. In one of his conversations he said,
"One primrose speaks of heaven, that is, the spirit; . . . . two
primroses speak of earth, that is, the manifest kingdom that
shows forth the spirit." The human being brings heaven and
earth to completion, brings together the heaven, the essence
of primrose, with the earth. On earth the many primroses are
propagated and nourished, all manifesting the One primrose. The call to life is the spirit, and the response to the call
to life is the manifest kingdom, the myriad expressions of
life, the One in the many.*

Each of us will show ourselves as the dance of heaven and
earth, as godly and earthly, as divine inspiration and as daily
breath, as one primrose and two primroses. We are continually completing the dance. You will recognize the whole of
me, the heaven and the earth of me in my laughter and song,
my shouting, weeping, moaning. You will know me through
my joy and compassion, my grief and fear and anger. We
will be all the elements to one another. We are the no-one,
anyone, someone, everyone self, all in One.

You are me. I am you. This is the basis for saying that
healing is not just a personal private event. Healing is a
transpersonal public event, a homecoming for all of us when
anyone comes home. We are "great oneness." The great life
force flows within you, within me, between us, among us.
We are guided by generations, beckoning, summoning, calling to one another—children together, comforters, guides,

---

*Within the framework of acupuncture, I suggest that the Governor Vessel (*du mo*)
may be viewed as the call to life, and the Conception Vessel (*ren mo*) as the
response to the call to life.

companions, from our personal and beyond our personal abilities. We get tired and raggedy. We go beyond our own raggedy tiredness. Everything comes up, both the useless and useful. Life occurs and occurs. There is nothing that is not an acknowledgment of being here in life, of being enveloped by life, lived by life. We are home, here between heaven and earth, ever on the circle, navigating the territory of survival and creation, the personal and the nonpersonal. In the personal I am distinct from you, and you from me. In the nonpersonal we are indistinguishable from each other.

The practitioner of traditional acupuncture in being with her patient dances between the personal and the nonpersonal. I am reminded of Catherine in *Wuthering Heights* when she exclaims: "I am Heathcliff." Of course, she is not Heathcliff in the sense of looking like him or having the personal detail of him, yet we know what she means. We all recognize the dance of her claim. In another story—"Tale from Attar" of Nishapur—a lover knocks on the door of his beloved. "Who knocks?" said the beloved from within. "It is I," said the lover. "Go away. This house will not hold you and me." The rejected lover went away into the desert. There he meditated for months on end, pondering the words of the beloved. Finally, he returned and knocked at the door again. "Who knocks?"—"It is you." The door was immediately opened.

Yet another expression of this theme is in the following quote from Teilhard de Chardin's *Hymn of the Universe*. I give it in its entirety because I think that it states profoundly the essence of this chapter and the conversation that the great healing art of acupuncture makes possible:

> Only love can bring individual beings to their perfect completion, as individuals, by uniting them one with another, because only love takes possession of them and unites them by what lies deepest within them. This is simply a fact of our everyday experience. For indeed at what moment do lovers come into the most complete possession of themselves if not

when they say they are lost in one another? And is not love all the time achieving—in couples, in teams, all around us—the magical and reputedly contradictory feat of personalizing through totalizing? And why should not what is thus daily achieved on a small scale be repeated one day on world-wide dimensions?

Humanity, the spirit of the earth, the synthesis of individuals and peoples, the paradoxical conciliation of the element with the whole, of the one with the many: all these are regarded as utopian fantasies, yet they are biologically necessary; and if we could see them made flesh in the world what more need we do than imagine our power to love growing and broadening till it can embrace the totality of humanity and of the earth?

Could it be that what widens within us forever is the ongoing act of transformation that we call love, and sometimes give other names to, like healing, wholing, coming home? Could it be that the gift of life, at once impersonal and personal—impersonal inspiration and personal manifestation—is what unites us and grants us greatness, is what sanctifies our humanity? We live life embracing and hallowing. Acupuncture treatment is an embracing and hallowing. It opens to, widens to, the promise that life is. In the personalness of each life is Life, just as in the personalness of each ocean wave is Ocean. There are billions of human lives to be embraced, each a parable of humanity, each a homing, a responding to Life itself calling. And, in the life calling that we say is death, a beyond which we can not get, may be the remerging of personal life into Life. "The nothingness from which we came is our true home, from which we can not stray for long." (Lieh Tzu) It may be that how we recognize each other along our journey is the unspeakable Life we share at the heart of our speakable individual lifes.

"What is a friend?"—"Another I."

— Zeno

> Always search for your innermost nature in those
> you are with . . . .
>
> — Rumi

In Arthur Miller's *After the Fall*, there is a passage where Quentin asks Holga a question (this is after the holocaust) and she responds to his searchings:

QUENTIN. . . . . How did you get so purposeful, Holga? You're so full of joy and hope!

HOLGA. Quentin, I think it's a mistake to ever look for hope outside one's self. One day the house smells of fresh bread, the next of smoke and blood. One day you faint because the gardener cut his finger off, within a week you're climbing over the corpses of children bombed in a subway. What hope can there be if that is so? I tried to die near the end of the war . . . . The same dream returned each night until I dared not go to sleep and grew quite ill. I dreamed I had a child, and even in the dream I saw it was my life, and it was an idiot, and I ran away. But it always crept onto my lap again, clutched at my clothes. Until I thought, if I could kiss it, whatever in it was my own, perhaps I could sleep. And I bent to its broken face, and it was horrible . . . . but I kissed it. I think one must finally take one's life in one's arms, Quentin . . . .

The embrace, the perpetual taking of one's life in one's arms no matter what it looks like, the reconciliation of all of the parts into one whole, the homecoming, the union of the personal with the cosmic—these are the purpose of the traditional acupuncture examination and treatment. The call to life is from Life itself, our ground of being. Life is who we are. We are more than beckoned. We are summoned to embrace it as it shows up in our individual self, our community self, our global self. Together we receive the mighty clarion. Together we respond to the call, and thus it is we lead each other home.

114

Life as interpreted by the five great movements of life—
Fire, Earth, Metal, Water, Wood—the Five Elements, the
Wu Hsing cycle, is embraced and expressed in the following
passage I wrote in 1974, three weeks before giving birth to
my son Blaize. I include it here in the chapter "Great Oneness" as an illustration of the personal-nonpersonal dance
that we are forever dancing, as the completion of heaven-
earth, one primrose-two primroses that life "is."

THE FIVE ELEMENTS —
REFLECTIONS BEFORE BIRTH:

Dear Baby beneath my heart. I write this to you while you
are in my belly. What I know about you is that you are
Nature—the elements so mixed in harmony—blended in
balance—simple mysteries. I am united with you forever,
though soon you will leave me.

> How do I know the ways of all things
>   at the Beginning?
> By what is within me.

> — Lao Tze

Earth: In the centre of me—in my earth—rich and fertile
you are nourished. I feel your touch from the inside and I am
fed. We sing together the hymn of the universe.

> You can not put a fence around the planet earth.
> I am the land. I wait.

> — O. Ortiz

> from spiralling ecstatically this

> proud nowhere of earth's most prodigious night
> blossoms a newborn babe . . .
> . . . .
> mind without doubt may blast some universe

115

to might have been,and stop ten thousand stars
but not one heartbeat of this child;nor shall
even prevail a million questionings
against the silence of his mother's smile

—whose only secret all creation sings

— ee cummings

Metal: I breathe and heaven pulses through you—and me. It is this breath that binds you to life, that carries you into life—whole, pure, rich—jewel of life's longing for itself . . . . taking in and letting go forever.

Kiss me, my father,
Touch me with your lips as I touch those I love,
Breathe to me while I hold you close the secret of
the murmuring . . . .

— Walt Whitman

Water: You move fluid within fluid—waters fed by the streams of humanity—waters that bathe your path from my body to the world. You are a river of life—sparkling, clear, forceful in your rhythmic flow.

Here are the waters and your watering place.
Drink and be whole again beyond confusion.

— Robert Frost

You, like a rivulet swift and sinuous, laugh and
dance, and your steps sing as you trip along.
I, like a bank rugged and steep, stand speechless
and stockstill and darkly gaze at you . . . .

— Rabindranath Tagore

Wood: You are springtime—alive and growing—tender sweet young sapling empowering us all to be born. We touch in our roots.

The trembling leaves of this tree touch my heart
like the fingers of an infant child.

— Rabindranath Tagore

I want
to do with you what spring does with the cherry
trees.

— Pablo Neruda

Fire: The sun shines the length of you, and the depth. You are warm in your cosmic sac sparked by the fire of loins' passionate communion. The summer is you—sweet succulent fruit held in the brown roundness of my belly. It is time for you to come now.

How far are you from me, O Fruit?
I am hidden in your heart, O Flower.

— Rabindranath Tagore

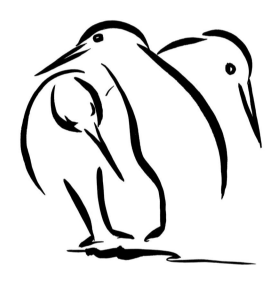

Who Is Home?

CHAPTER ELEVEN

Who Is Home?

(To patients)

Is there anything left on which late-twentieth-century man can build if he is to seek a homecoming to the house of being?

— Martin Heidegger

What is known I strip away,
I launch all men and women forward with me into the Unknown.

— Walt Whitman

We need a place to tell our stories . . . . democracy was created to make the world safe for telling stories.

— Hannah Arendt

Twenty men crossing a bridge,
Into a village,
Are twenty men crossing twenty bridges
Into twenty villages,
Or one man
Crossing a single bridge into a village.

— Wallace Stevens

your homecoming will be my homecoming

— ee cummings

. . . . Novalis said: "Philosophy . . . . is strictly speaking a homesickness."

It is not a discipline that can be learned. The sciences are only servants in relation to it. But art and religion are its sisters. He who does not know what homesickness is, cannot philosophize. It is only possible for us to philosophize if, and because, we do not feel at home anywhere, because we are unceasingly being pushed up against Being, against that in Being which is total and essential, because we feel at home nowhere except on the way to total and essential. We are without a native land and are restlessness itself, living restlessness: it is because of *this* that it is necessary for us to philosophize. And this restlessness is *our* confinement, in us who are finitude itself. And we are not allowed to let it pass away, to comfort ourselves in an illusion about totality and a satisfactory infinitude. We must not only bear [this restlessness] in us, but accentuate it, and when we are not only confined but entirely isolated, only then do we strive more to incite ourselves to be important, civilized; only then are we in a position to be "gripped."

And when we thus make ourselves grippable, by handing ourselves over to reality, our homesickness makes us into human beings.

— Martin Heidegger

It would be very good if we would wake up before we die.

— Old Hindu Saying

H arry's mother calls him to get up for school. The conversation goes as follows: "O Ma, do I have to?" "Yes, Harry, you have to. Come on now and get up. It's a school day." "Aw, Ma." "Harry." "Ma, give me two good reasons why I

122

have to get up and go to school." "Well, first of all, Harry, you are forty-five years old, and secondly, you're the principal!"

Ma *and* Harry am I. "Come on, Dianne, you have things to be about." "Aw, Dianne, do I have to take this journey?" "Yes. Yes. Yes. It is time now, and you are responsible for your life."

So, here I am, forty-one years old, full of my life, aware of my history, my pains, my turning points, my joys, my touch-stones. My heart is beating. My blood is flowing. I am a mother of two children, Blaize and Jade. I teach. I write. I have been a practitioner of traditional acupuncture for fif-teen years now. I am a woman. I have my story, all the chapters and vignettes. I still need a mother, a guide who reminds me to wake up, to get up. I am a traveling companion.

And even as I am here looking into the who-I-am, I look at you, reader, like a waiting lover . . . . full of your life, knowing and not knowing yourself . . . . open to me, to my life, to our life together.

> I celebrate myself, and sing myself,
> And what I assume you shall assume,
> For every atom belonging to me as good belongs
>   to you.
>
> — Walt Whitman

We are all members of the human family, children on the planet Earth. We are brothers and sisters lost and found often along our way. We seek to know the face of our love, the nature of who we are, and the home that life is. We want to be known, to be understood, to be called out of hiding. I write reaching into your life, the center of me to the center of you, gathering myself to give to you . . . knowing that is all we really have or want from one another. I am somewhere on the circle, in the cycle of nature at every moment. So are you. Find me. Find you. I am calling out like Tommy, the blind, deaf, dumb, pinball machine wizard: "See me, feel me, touch me, heal me." I am saying who I am, who I think myself to be, who I think you think I am. Listen to my voice—the words and the music. Look at me with your eyes wide open, all of your eyes, the whole of your sight. Watch me live. Talk to me, searching my nooks and my crannies with a promise to know me in ways I do not yet know. Touch me, molecule to molecule, thought to thought, feeling to feeling, heart to heart. Go the length of me. Plumb my depths. Come home with me.

Two-thirds of the way through a traditional acupuncture examination, a young male patient, Casey, said to me ever so quietly, nearly whispering. "Both my parents are deaf." In the hush of his speaking we were both listening intently. Together we could see how his life was the living of the question, "Do you hear me?" It was his leitmotiv. It was here he suffered. All of his symptoms, i.e., his inability to concentrate, to focus on his work, problems with drink, fear of intimacy with women, flashes of uncontrollable anger—all were ways of getting himself heard, all were situations that in the very process of living made clear his internal dilemma. Rumi, the Sufi poet, said, "If you've not been fed, be bread." Casey continually gives his listening to his friends, knowing the power of being heard even in the face of his own personal struggle to make himself heard. When asked what his friends count on him for, he realized in astonishment that they come to him for his willingness and capacity to hear them.

This is the wisdom of illness. It is a call to come home to the ground of being. All sickness is homesickness, homesick for ourselves and for each other. All our daily events, events born of the day, are our journey manifest, our call to come home. All healing is a coming home. The journey is a cycle, a circle of movement, the great *Wu-Hsing*, the five great movements of nature: the Fire that warms and burns, the Earth that nourishes and starves, the Metal that gives breath and takes it away, the Water that flows and runs dry, the

124

Wood that grows and gets old. And so we go—we'll laugh together and sing and weep and groan and shout. We'll be joyful and compassionate and grieving and fearful and angry. We are everonthecircle: labyrinth . . . . wilderness . . . . clearing . . . . mountain . . . . valley . . . . hardpatch . . . . easypatch . . . . storm . . . . calm . . . . river . . . . wind . . . . garden . . . . desert . . . . pond . . . . stream . . . . season to season . . . . day to day . . . . hour to hour . . . . moment to moment . . . . "The wonders we seek are within us."

We *will* know our wonder as a person, a people, a planet. We *are* the Journey. We *are* Home. Our collective bond is the force of life itself.

What goes on in the treatment room is a tapping of life as an empowering event. Traditional acupuncture is a system of healing that looks to all of a person and sees the entirety of the individual as an expression of Ch'i, the life force, the essence of life manifesting. Nothing of a person's life is judged bad or good, it simply is. Everything is seen and held simply as an expression of the person en route to knowing who she is, self reaching for self. Everything in each human's life is seen as an integrated picture consistent with her journey. Health is a dynamic experience of this integrity, no matter what the circumstances of the daily life, the tasks at hand at the moment—diapering the baby, putting in the needle, delivering a lecture, making love, washing dishes, praying. As she taps the power of being in her own life, it is as though she has swallowed a hand grenade with the pin pulled out, and in slow motion begins to realize what she has done: an internal explosion occurs, and though she may look like her old self in appearance, a transformation happens from which she will not recover, nor will she want to. In the awesome recognition of her homecoming, in the irrevocable acknowledgment of her Nature, she is no longer estranged from herself. Every estrangement henceforth will point her homeward.

It is through our Nature that we master our symptoms, that we break through habits and patterns that no longer serve us, that we change the ways that have ceased to be useful in our lives. We shift from being possessed by our history and all its content to being in command of our own homecoming. "I am more at home in myself. I have a grasp on my struggles.—I can use them. If a headache starts, I don't automatically dread it. I'm calmer now." These are words of a person beginning to recognize her power to be healthy. This is a shift from a position of being the victim of a symptom, to being in balance and harmony in relation to the symptom. From here the patient begins to gain her whole life, seeing herself in the world, both her internal and external world, as a creative force. She grows to trust her own life, to observe the varied expressions of herself—gestures, thoughts, interactions, reactions, patterns of eating, sleeping, emotions, upsets, symptoms; to see the relationships and watch the tapestry she weaves in a day's time, not as a voyeur, but as a voyager in the kingdom of self. She opens to all of life, and gives thanks. She realizes that her task is the same as the task of every human being—to be home in her self, to live her life fully and authentically, knowing she is not here alone nor only for herself. She is here for life, shepherdess for the homecoming of human being.

Who comes for treatment, what brings them, what is the heart of their story, what is my challenge with them . . . .

> . . . . uniqueness gives interpenetration its dynamism—without it, there would be no Chinese, as distinguished from the Norwegian, to be one with the Norwegian.
>
> — Robert Aiken

Although this chapter is addressed to patients—the who of who is home—its purpose is to illustrate that each of us is a portrait of life itself, each of us is the dance visited upon itself, life taking us. I see this dance, the portrayal of life living itself, most profoundly in the treatment room—yet I assume that it occurs anywhere there is human being.

The following are ten profiles of patients who have been examined and treated. Each highlights some fundamental of healing, each points out the uniqueness and complexity of every single person, while at the same time pointing to a simplicity and unity that binds us all.

Nan is a woman, age thirty-four, a pharmacist, who comes for treatment because of sinus headaches, which, she says, "keep me from feeling that my head belongs to me." Recently married, she says that she is "unable to enjoy myself and my husband sexually." She cried during the examination, a deep sobbing with no holding back, when I asked her about her childhood. She recalled an incident when she was eight years old of witnessing a car accident in which the driver's head smashed through the windshield and was gushing blood. In recounting the story, Nan realized that she ran and hid and never said anything to anybody about what she had seen, and that she had nightmares of blood gushing from her own head; when she got her period for the first time and saw the blood gushing, she also ran and hid, keeping it to herself. She then wondered whether her sinus headaches and her sexual holding back were "hideouts" from letting her life gush forth now. Nan is a wonderful example of people making brand new and freeing connections as they inquire into the already familiar territory of their life. What is empowering is not so much the particular insights, which of course are exciting to her, but the opening to inquire again and again to continually create new openings for her life, to reveal her own possibilities. Nan and I work well together. She is willing to grapple with hard issues and use me as her guide. I have been treating her in Fire, especially the Three-Heater and Circulation-Sex. She reports being outgoing now, having fun in sex and playing with her husband in lots of new ways. Just before her period her head aches sometimes, but she knows it's her head and belongs to her. She is home with herself.

Steve is a man, forty-one years old, a carpenter who suffers with low back pain and who began treatment when his western physician recommended that he have surgery to fuse part of his lumbar spine. This man suffers emotionally as well. His nine-year-old son is deaf. Steve blamed himself. From where he was looking, he was missing his son and didn't know it. I could hear that his story, his "because" about his son's deafness, was keeping him unavailable to his child. I could also hear that his back was a manifestation of the burden he carried. He was caught in an interpretation of a circumstance that he could not see beyond. He, to himself, was unequivocally the cause of his son's deafness, even though it was not reasonable. From where he was listening, he could not get home to himself, or his son. We started treatment. We began in the Wood Element. After the first treatment, he got "fiercely angry with God," which he experienced as a relief of personal guilt. For the second treatment I used the source point in Wood called "Wilderness Mound." Right after the needle, Steve sat upright as though he had felt something powerful and he said, "I must forgive my humanness, my son his deafness." I thought of the words of Dag Hammarskjöld in *Markings*, "Forgiveness breaks the chain of causality . . . ." Steve was healing. He was responding to the call from Life to life, the call he had not heard before. He was forgiving, breaking the chain of causality. He was coming home. His son was waiting for him.

Will is a man, eighty years old, beloved father of three children and grandfather of four. We fell for each other immediately. He told me how Mark Twain toward the end of his life said, "I'm an old man now and I've had lots of troubles, half of which never happened. Don't worry. Don't hurry. Smell the roses along the way." This man's way of being is a clear example of living life right on the edge of one's seat. He came for treatment because one of his daughters had told him how wonderful it was for her, so he figured it would be great for him too. It is a whole new way for him to look at his health. He said, "I see the possibility of serenity. I could use a little help with that, and who knows what else." For Will, the Earth Element is his most crucial support. The

Earth is the great cradle that holds all of life, that has room
for the daisy and the weed, the yes and the no, the robin
and the wolf, the poet and the scientist, the gain and the
loss, the wound and the gift. It is the promise of home for all
in the cycle of life. Will has been in the cycle, on the circle,
for longer than most of us. He knows that the storyteller is
not the story, and that life is bigger and more mysterious than
any interpretation of it. In the evening of the day I first met
Will I returned home after work and there waiting for me
was a most beautiful green growing plant and a note that
said, "Oh to be forty-five again!" I quickly sent a note back to
him saying: "Oh to be seventy-five anon!" (He is eighty!)
Will exemplifies the great joy in life, the joy of being alive
every minute, living it all, no matter what's coming next or
what happened before. Being home in life.

Jimmy is a baby boy, nine months old, who was born
prematurely. When he was born he appeared to be not fully
arrived—he was slow in responding to stimulus, and was not
growing at the same rate as other babies his age. His mother
is a friend of someone I treat, so she asked to bring him for
treatment. It is not usual to treat one so small, but when it
looked like he could be served well, I chose to treat him. For
six months now I have been treating Jimmy in the Water
Element. His mother and I both observe that Jimmy is completing his delivery and birth. He is stronger, more fiery,
more available; he laughs more, has more movement of his
arms and legs, more expression of himself. Though it is
difficult to prognose the pattern and pace of his continued
arrival, Jimmy is most certainly coming home to himself, his
mother, his whole family—his progress is also verified by
western medical tests. No matter what our age we yearn to
be home.

Kate is a woman, sixty years old, a housewife who is
looking after her aging mother. She lives, not to relieve the
tensions of the day, but to create home as a way of being, as a
constant opening to life, life with all name and no name, with
face of all and no face, the home that is like the one the

Brazilians say we have a homesickness for, "Saldage," a place we know does not really exist, but that we know is really home. Kate described a moving moment: "I took my eighty-year-old mother's face in my hands and we looked into each other's eyes up close. My mother spoke: "There is one face." Kate comes for treatment because she has high blood pressure, because it is not easy for her to take care of her mother and because she is anxious about her own aging and dying. Treatment in the Metal Element is a most powerful life support for Kate. She is inspirational in her commitment to the quality of life for everyone around her, and she requires the strength to keep letting go and emptying herself of expectations of what life "should" look like. When we have no expectations, we are home where we are. We are empty vessels.

> home means that
> when the certainly
> roof leaks it
> 's our(home
>
> means if any moon
> or possibly
> sun shines they are
> our also my
>
> darling) . . . .
>
> — ee cummings

Philip is a man, twenty years old, who wrestles. As he says, "I became a wrestler to overcome my feelings of inadequacy as a kid." He comes for treatment because of injuries and places where his body continues to hurt—his back in several places, his knees, his left shoulder. He is in a relationship and afraid he's "going to blow it." "I don't trust anyone." Philip has always been looking for himself. He is like the Zen picture of the oxherd, sitting on an ox looking for the ox. His whole life has been to look for his life, thereby missing the experience of being present to himself. Yet, to be with him you would say he is *life itself* manifesting, and you would trust him. His strength and his struggle emerge from the same source. I treat Philip primarily in Wood.

Janie is thirteen years old, about to have her period, looking forward to it and being terrified at the same time. She is coming into the flower of young womanhood. She is afraid of being boring, of not "measuring up," and being disapproved of by her friends. Janie is asking questions like, Who am I? What is life about? Am I capable? Who is my mother to me? Who is my father to me?—a thirteen-year-old human being asking questions from her young bodymindspirit. Sometimes she calls me up to ask whether I've ever felt the way she feels. When she comes for treatment, she is mostly asking for strength and support, particularly in Earth so that she knows that she's got her own ground to stand on, that she can count on herself, and that the questions she has—Will people like me? Am I boring?—are questions that are an inverted looking at her commitment to be present to other people, to be interested in life, and to be a measure for all that life will open her to. Treatment acts as a kind of pivot for Janie, a reference point for her to keep returning home to herself.

George is a man, fifty years old, chief executive of a large corporation. He has a big vision for what may be possible in the corporate world. He comes for treatment because he gets migraine headaches and because he experiences treatment as a sanctuary, a space for homing his daily events. He knows there are no answers for how to dwell in life, and he is intent on keeping with the powerful questions. He struggles in the intimate partnership with his wife. I treat him in Fire as the source and promise of light, of illumination, and of warmth and relationship. For George being a visionary at work is relatively easy, but being a visionary in his marriage is more difficult. He occasionally gets a headache now, but lately he has been using any hint of a headache as a good signal to be still.

> Teach us to care and not to care
> Teach us to sit still
> Even among these rocks . . . .

— T. S. Eliot

Sally is a woman, age thirty-one, an actress of great beauty and depth. She "died" in an airplane crash when she was twenty-five. She had no heartbeat, and then she revived, becoming the only survivor among fourteen people. Her main reason for treatment is her experience of different parts of her "going dead, a kind of paralysis roaming her body compounded by extreme vertigo." Sally loves acting as a way of exploring and expressing the depths of humanity. She reminded me of the words from the Upanishads: "If you want the Truth as badly as a drowning person wants air, you will realize it in a moment." This young woman lives her life courageously and acts on stage as though her life depends on it. Maybe it does. Maybe that is the power of our actions— our life is at stake. I treat Sally via the Water Element, especially the Kidney, the "Storehouse of the Vital Essence." She responds quickly, like a thirsty person with a drink of water. The original complaint that brought her in the door is gone. Only occasionally now does she have vertigo. She told me the other day that she is in awe most of the time, moved by life, glad to be alive. Sally is a continual wake-up call to me, to all of us, her fellow travelers.

Tom is a man, thirty-six years old, doctor of internal medicine. He lives with a man, his love, who has been diagnosed as having Acquired Immunodeficiency Syndrome. Both of them are scared. Their prevailing conversation about the illness is that the disease is bigger than they are, and that there is no possibility of altering it or themselves. Much of Tom's dialogue with me is directed toward the unsayable, the mystery of illness and death. As he reaches to make sense of his circumstances, he comes up against his own frailty, insecurity, mortality, humanity. The only place he can go is straight into his suffering for the possibility of freedom. I am reminded of Marcel Proust's statement, "We are healed of a suffering only by experiencing it to the full," and Lao Tze's, ". . . . equipped with this timeless Tao, you can harness present realities." I treat Tom in Metal, the great movement in nature of taking in the pure Ch'i from the heavens and the letting go of all that no longer serves our human life, and eventually letting go of everything, releasing in the end the very breath that heralded the entering of "I" at birth. It is not easy for Tom, nor for his love, nor for me, to face the most awesome of mysteries, the transformation of life in death, and yet, we must as an expression of authentic being. We can assign neither our dying nor our living to one another. We must present ourselves.

> Let us always love one another, and so forgive one another for appearing, for changing, and for passing out of present sight. So be it.
>
> — Da Free John

There are many others who come for treatment:

Josie, a twenty-nine-year-old black poetess who is afraid of the "voice that is great within" her; Susie, a five-year-old with breathing difficulties, at whose birth I was present; Cynthia, a seventy-six-year-old philosopher who had cancer twenty-eight years ago, and who maintains her life by continually giving it away; David, a forty-two-year-old high school teacher, whose life promise is to bring kids forth to their own lives, teaching them to express themselves; Dirk, fifty-three, a former CIA agent who became a gardener; Peter, fifteen, in high school and unhappy with what he experiences as pressure; Barbara, thirty-nine years old, five-months pregnant with her first baby. The Great Human Company, bearing witness to its humanity, listening through to the godliness. ". . . . for the god wants to know himself in you." (Rilke)

Heidegger says that "poetry is the saying of the unconcealedness of beings, ... the saying of world and earth, the saying of the arena of their strife and thus of the place of all nearness and remoteness of the gods." When we human beings speak our symptoms, there is a kind of poetry, an unconcealing of life. Pain calls us to life, to the who that speaks the pain, to the one who says the sayable.

> when the traveler returns from the mountain-slopes into the
>   valley,
> he brings, not a handful of earth, unsayable to others, but
>   instead
> some word he has gained, some pure word, the yellow and
>   blue
> gentian. Perhaps we are here in order to say: house,
> bridge, fountain, gate, pitcher, fruit-tree, window—
>   . . . .
> *Here* is the time for the *sayable, here* is its homeland. Speak
> and bear witness . . . .
>
> — Rainer Maria Rilke

> until out of merely not nothing comes
> only one snowflake (and we speak our names)
>
> — ee cummings

The sayable and the unsayable stand side by side in the day, in our ordinary space and time. When human beings speak they open up what is not spoken; as we name things and ourselves, life which has no name, appears. As practitioner and patient attend to the Life beyond what is named in the treatment room, they find their way home—and know they have been there always.

> Being's poem, just begun, is man.
>
> — Martin Heidegger

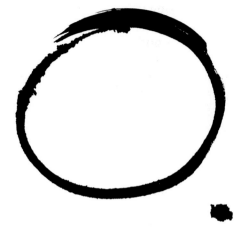

萬
物

As is, No Matter What

CHAPTER TWELVE

As Is, No Matter What

Fare forward, you who think that you are voyaging;
· · · · · · · · · ·

At the moment which is not of action or inaction
You can receive this: "on whatever sphere of being
The mind of a man may be intent
At the time of death"—that is the one action
(And the time of death is every moment)
Which shall fructify in the lives of others:
· · · · · · · · · ·
Fare forward.

— T. S. Eliot

When the sun rises
I go to work
When the sun goes down
I take my rest
I share creation
Kings can do no more.

— Ancient Chinese Saying

Not long ago, in the evening, I was driving my red Checker along an unfamiliar country road. I was heading for a place I had never been before, so I had a map but no acquaintance with the territory itself. The darker it got, the more afraid I became about not getting to my destination, and even worse, not finding my way back home either. I started to panic with my full-scale life-symphony of "lost" in the background: all the remembrances of childhood and being away from home and unsure about getting there again played their strains. Incidents kept coming to mind of other times and places. People whom I cherish entered this internal dialogue. I could see how much my life is about lost and found. I could see how precious my loves are to me. I could see that when I am by myself I am not alone. Then, in the midst of this lostness, it occurred to me: "Suppose I'm okay. Suppose it is not possible to be lost, and that feeling lost is simply an interpretation of how I do not know where I am. Suppose, Dianne, that you are right here where you are. You've been doing all this fancy talk about being home, that everything is a call to come home to yourself, well then, what's this lostness? Suppose you are already home and that this is what it looks like now. Suppose there is no place to get to, and only a place to come from every moment. Suppose confusion is only a clutching for an answer. Suppose you are always home? Suppose that 'coming from home' is not about a chronological time and geographic place called home as much as it is a speaking of the promise underlying the whole of life, that is, wherever I am, home is. If I am home you can be home with me. Suppose I am home." In this conversation my fear died. I was on "home base." I located the house I had been searching for. And, later, I made it back to my house just fine.

This is a telling vignette. The theme of lostness comes up in human life. Telling one's story can open up the home inherent in lostness. In the treatment room, in the midst of a lot of story and circumstance of a person's life, it is rather easy to get lost, that is, to forget that the story and circumstance are expressing home, pointing toward home, calling us homeward, and not something in themselves significant, or for the sake of themselves. Suppose the patient is home, as is. I mean it, as is, with all of her history, complaints, struggles, as is, with nothing changed.

Suppose we are already home and this is what home looks like.

Suppose we are not lost and that we are never lost, really.

Suppose we are in promise to love one another as is, no matter what, and that is our fundamental nature.

Suppose we have gotten who we are, and forgotten.

Suppose every upset is a call to come home, to be home, to be at home.

Suppose everything we don't like and everything we do like equally point us homeward.

Suppose we really matter to one another.

Suppose my life is yours, yours mine.

Suppose I give my life to you.

Suppose every moment is a gift no matter how it appears.

If she is already home *as is*, how do I interact with my patient? What is the nature of our relationship if I see her as already whole? What sort of work do we do together? What does it look like? The following is an example of working in wholeness. It is a sharing of someone who moved me deeply being exactly herself, as she was, no matter what. This is my "Hymn to Charlotte."

Charlotte gave me life even as she was dying. She called me awake over and over again. I share her with you as a gift, just as she was a gift to me. She came to me for treatment having been diagnosed as having breast cancer. She was thirty-eight years old, a woman with deep and abiding wisdom. She used me in ways I did not even know I was useful. Because we were the same age, because she had two children as I do, because she was scared as I was, it seemed that my ability to support her life was surpassed by my personal considerations. I wanted to run away, to not see her surgerized, chemotherapied body, to not engage in those conversations about death and life, to not assist her in letting go of her life as we both had known it, to not be with her in her ultimate reckoning with her self; and yet, I did not run. She held me steady. She taught me how to be with her, how to guide her, how to see her and support her to the very ends of her being, to the very end of her life.—Dianne, see me; be with me; navigate this new uncharted territory with me; don't let anything come between us, not the emaciation, not the disorientation, not even the pain. Partner me in this passage—no matter how rough. Charlotte, I can't. Yes, you can, Dianne; be with me, and be with me in the hour of my death. She guided me the whole route.

She loved coming to the Centre for Traditional Acupuncture. It was home to her. Everyone engaged with her and she drew us together as family, not from sympathy, but from a celebration of life. She died during the hours of the Great Letting Go, according to the Chinese body clock, the time of Metal (3 a.m. - 7 a.m.). Most of the treatments I had given her were to support her Earth and Metal, the dance of Earth and Heaven, of Mother and Father in every human being. Weeks before she died Charlotte had come to peace with her earthly mother after years of struggle. And, a most amazing event happened two hours before she died: a night nurse was singing and teaching me to sing Negro spirituals there at the bedside where Charlotte lay in a coma in the hospital, when in came two young men looking rather unkempt. One of them said he was Charlotte's half brother by the same father, and that their father was away somewhere on holiday and could not be reached. Their father did not know she was dying, and this brother had not seen his sister for years. "I came to tell Charlotte I love her." He then went over to her, laid his hand upon hers and began to pray, "Our Father, Who art in Heaven. Hallowed be Thy Name. Thy Kingdom come. Thy will be done on Earth as it is in Heaven . . . ."

The earth moved that night. O holy night. Charlotte died healing. She healed in her dying. We all healed in her dying.

She gave me myself by refusing to engage with me with anything less than herself. I think about her often, especially when I am in rough passage, what I call a "hard patch," and I hear "Come on, Dianne—if I can do this, you can do that." None of this conversation solves the mystery around and about death, the "whys" are no more uncovered. What is illuminated is how one person's life, one person's majesty in the face of the circumstance of death, no matter how awesome, called the rest of us to life, to what is of essence. She taught me about myself through herself; she called me to be with her, and therefore myself. Nothing is difficult for very long any more.

Charlotte, I thank you for my life. I thank you for showing me over and over that *as is* life is gift, *no matter what.*

COME, COME, WHOEVER YOU ARE
WANDERER, WORSHIPPER, LOVER OF LEAVING
IT DOESN'T MATTER.
OURS IS NOT A CARAVAN OF DESPAIR.
COME, EVEN IF YOU HAVE BROKEN YOUR VOW
    A THOUSAND TIMES.
COME, YET AGAIN, COME, COME.

— Sufi Poet

The conversation of this chapter peers into life inclusive of suffering and death. Not for nothing. In his book *Who Dies?* Stephen Levine asserts, "We seldom use illness as an opportunity to investigate our relationship to life or to explore our fear of death." Then, he asks, "How do we allow ourselves to come into the unknown with an openheartedness and courage that allow life its fullness?" He further asserts that "as long as we are thinking of healing as opposed to dying, there will be confusion."

Isn't it time to make room for illness, suffering and death? Isn't life the cradle in which we have come to know what we call dying? Does healing have to look any particular way?

Does it mean no symptoms, no pains, no undergoing and going-through of unknown experiences, no death? If we posit healing in opposition to death, and I would also say, in opposition to illness, then we live in the mode of defending and protecting ourselves from dying and hurting. Then we are in a fight and running a really risky business of not living fully alive. It may be that we are suffering when we are not fully alive. If that be so, then suffering becomes an experience calling us to the fullness of life, calling us to being, calling us home.

Perhaps holding illness, disease, suffering as bad and fighting them, that is, being opposed to them, and attempting to get rid of them as though they do not belong to life, obscures the possibility of embracing that which may point us homeward, that which maybe in the end bears us home to our beginning, to the source from whence we have come. With no fixed ideas about what healing should look like, we can open beyond struggle, beyond the interpretation of suffering-symptom as enemy. It may be that resistance to pain makes the pain persist—not that we should love the pain, but perhaps, somehow we could embrace it as a calling from life, as an expression of being. To heal one must be prepared to die, to surrender to being wherever that may take us. Healing and dying fabricate the same opening, call on the same listening of life, the same attention to being.

During the months before she died, my patient Bonnie used her pain like a drill master, an instructor. When she felt a wave of sharp constriction in her chest, she would come to attention, absolutely still and alert, expecting nothing, listening to what she described as "babies breathing." Her presence in those moments was so total, so unencumbered, so free. She was pure being, doing nothing. Oh to have life as she had it in her dying! Bonnie's death was a complete action of her being. The whole power of her self was required for dying.

Nothing is more creative than death, since it is the whole secret of life. It means that the past must be abandoned, that the unknown can not be avoided, that "I" can not continue and that nothing can be ultimately fixed.

— Alan Watts

We think we know what death is. We even think we know what illness is, or if not know now, then ultimately we can know sometime, with enough research and study. However, if I return my entire life to the domain of not knowing, then everything, instead of being something I already know becomes alive again and new and possible, becomes creation. In the light of newly possible, illness and death become phenomena to inquire about, not for answers to solve the mystery once and for all, but for a glimmering of the nature of who we are and what we are doing here on the planet Earth.

The following are human speakings of that which is "sayable" about death, and therefore about life.

From all the rest I single out you, having a message for you,
You are to die—let others tell you what they please, I cannot
    prevaricate,
I am exact and merciless, but I love you—there is no escape
    for you.

Softly I lay my right hand upon you, you just feel it,
I do not argue, I bend my head close and half envelop it,
I sit quietly by, I remain faithful,
I am more than nurse, more than parent or neighbor,
I absolve you from all except yourself spiritual bodily,
    that is eternal,
        you yourself will surely escape,
The corpse you will leave will be but excrementitious.

The sun bursts through in unlooked-for directions,
Strong thoughts fill you and confidence, you smile,
You forget you are sick, as I forget you are sick,

You do not see the medicines, you do not mind the weeping
    friends,
        I am with you,
I exclude others from you, there is nothing to be
    commiserated,
I do not commiserate, I congratulate you.

                      — Walt Whitman

O I see now that life cannot exhibit all to me, as
    the day cannot,
I see that I am to wait for what will be exhibited
    by death.

                      — Walt Whitman

    But Love has pitched his mansion in
    The place of excrement
    For nothing can be sole or whole
    That has not been rent

              — William Butler Yeats

Whatever I had I chose to have, obliging myself only to
possess it totally, and to taste the experience to the full. Thus
the most dreary tasks were accomplished with ease as long as
I was willing to give myself to them. Whenever an object
repelled me, I made it a subject of study, ingeniously compelling myself to extract from it a motive for enjoyment. If
faced with something unforeseen or near cause for despair,
like an ambush or a storm at sea, after all measures of safety
for the others had been taken, I strove to welcome this
hazard, to rejoice in whatever it brought me of the new and
unexpected, and thus without shock the ambush or the temp-
est was incorporated into my plans, or my thoughts. Even in
the throes of my worst disaster, I have seen a moment when
sheer exhaustion reduced some part of the horror of the
experience, and when I made the defeat a thing of my own in
being willing to accept it. If ever I am to undergo torture (and
illness will no doubt see to that) I cannot be sure of maintain-
ing the impassiveness of a Thrasea, but I shall at least have the

resource of resigning myself to my cries. And it is in such a way, with a mixture of reserve and daring, of submission and revolt carefully concerted, of extreme demand and prudent concession, that I finally learned to accept myself.

— Marguerite Yourcenar

I must learn that we must die.

— Theodore Roethke

Our natures are the physicians of our diseases.

— Hippocrates

All interest in disease and death is only another expression of interest in life. Hold every moment sacred.

— Thomas Mann

. . . . it may matter deeply how we end so mysterious a thing as living.

— Florida Scott-Maxwell

[Regarding Socrates] . . . . His death sentence was announced to him. That instant he dies—for one who does not understand that the whole power of the spirit is required for dying, and that the hero always dies before he dies, that man will not get so very far with his conception of life.

— Søren Kierkegaard

You and I are pilgrims . . . . We go forward . . . . beyond the known . . . . We make the . . . . conscious offering . . . . we induce our thoughts, our feelings, our bodies, all that we are, to be nothing but the force that leads us toward emptiness. There is not a trace of emotion in the movement of life toward death, only the posture of that moment of encounter when death makes life overflow in us . . . .
"In the quiet of your being, 'feel the gushing of the fountain: Thou art That.'"

— Lizelle Reymond, quoting her
guide on a pilgrimage

145

Human suffering, the sum total of suffering poured out at each moment over the whole earth, is like an immeasurable ocean . . . . it is potential *energy*. Suffering holds within it, in extreme intensity, the ascensional force of the world . . . . If all those who suffer in the world were to unite their sufferings so that the pain of the world should become one single grand act of consciousness, ... of unification, would not this be one of the most exalted forms in which the mysterious work of creation could be manifested to our eyes?

— Teilhard De Chardin

. . . . Lord . . . . grant that *when my hour has come* I may recognize you under the appearances of every alien or hostile power that seems bent on destroying or dispossessing me. When the erosions of age begin to leave their mark on my body, and still more on my mind; when the ills that must diminish my life or put an end to it strike me down from without or grow up from within me; when I reach that painful moment at which I suddenly realize that I am a sick man or that I am growing old; above all at that final moment when I am losing hold on myself and becoming wholly passive in the hands of those great unknown forces which first formed me . . . . grant me, Lord, to understand that it is you . . . . who are painfully separating the fibres of my being so as to penetrate to the very marrow of my substance and draw me into yourself.

The more deeply and incurably my ills become engrained in my flesh, the more it may be you yourself that I am harbouring as a loving, active principle of purification and of liberation from possessiveness . . . .

. . . . to receive communion as I die is not sufficient: teach me to make a communion of death itself.

— Teilhard De Chardin

We live like knowers, striving toward absolute information, but death is a perfect insult that frustrates all knowing . . . . We are not knowing in our pondering over death. We are contemplating Mystery, the answerless Paradox of our living

existence. The death of an other and the death of "I" confound the whole spectacle and consolation of knowledge....
Death is the transformation of the knower.

— Da Free John

Postscript

---

how generous is that himself the sun . . . .
. . . .
(never a moment ceasing to begin
the mystery of day for someone's eyes)
. . . .
—we are himself's own self; his very him

— ee cummings

I trust all joy.

— Theodore Roethke

There are as many interpretations about how life works as there are human beings living it. We are in continuous explanation, the "whys" and the "how-comes," explicating and translating the way things *are* in the kingdom—in the kingdom of self: self as person, as family, as global village. Life lives us and we interpret it—yet life is uninterpretable. It translates only to and from itself, and continues to confound us in its mystery, as we keep rendering accounts. We are life interpreting Life. Probably forever.

The ancient Chinese understood life in particular ways, and in what I find to be empowering interpretations. Their rendering opens extraordinary accounts of human beings as one with nature, one with the world. "How I know about the world is by what is within me" says Lao Tze. In the observation of the design of nature, the passage of time—for example, in a day, a season, a life—shows itself as a pattern. The ways of nature are rhythmic and circuitous, count-on-able and capricious, impersonal and personal. In being conscious of our life we become conscious of One playing many different parts. The Chinese interpret the movement of the Ch'i in the human being as perpetual flowing of the life force in twelve main channels, like rivers, each functional in a particular way in the human kingdom of bodymindspirit. They are the ways of life, the openings to new possibilities. They are the traveling routes, the paths, of the life force. Each is embraced by one of the five great movements, one of the Five Elements. Each is correlated with physical organic functioning, as well as all other aspects of human functioning. Each is held as a family member crucial and inseparable from all the rest. Each is the most important function in the integrity of family paradox. Each has its own points for direct address to the Ch'i. Each is an empowering touchstone for getting present to life. Each is a road in sight of home. Each is an entire step in the whole of the dance.

To know the universe itself as a road, as many roads,
   roads for
      traveling souls.

                                — Walt Whitman

Pick up a blade of grass and all the worlds come with it.

                                  — Alan Watts

To me, one of the most powerful interpretations of life is contained in the preceding two sentences. In the Taoist view, everything is what it is in relation to all the others, and concepts can not explain the phenomenon that is life. Alan Watts says it well, "There is no way of putting a stream in a bucket or the wind in a bag." We can not capture the universe. We can only be in relationship to the whole of it as we arrive where we are. We can only enter upon the road that opens before us and know that we are home in every step, always arriving. It is not so farfetched then, to think that all the facets of life can be correlated, just as the Chinese so long ago claimed.

Let us now take up just one of the twelve family members, functions, pathways of the life force, as an elucidation of an empowering interpretation of how life works. Dr. Worsley calls the twelve, the Officials, the dignitaries of the kingdom, the kingdom of self—bodymindspirit. Manfred Porkert calls them orbs and refers to all twelve as "Orbisiconography," that is, "the comprehensive and systematic description of energetic processes taking place in the microcosm (i.e., within an individual organism) and of the dynamic relations that may be defined or postulated through empirical observation of these processes." Pere Claude Larre says that there really is no translation for the twelve, although he in one writing used the word "charges," meaning "ways to operate with a responsibility to the highest . . . . Heaven." These twelve are the organizing principles, the design of the creation—human being. As we take up one, we take up the family. As we take up one, we take up the human being. We take up humanity.

The Three-Heater. This family member, the Three-Heater, is held in the great movement of nature that we call Fire. It goes by other names too—*san-chiao, orbis tricalorii,* Three Burning Spaces, Triple Warmer, Three Heated Spaces. Here I will usually call it the Three-Heater. It is a function that has a name, yet it has no physical organ correlate, unlike, for example, the function named the Supreme Controller, whose physical organ correlate is the heart; or the function named Separator of Pure from Impure, whose anatomical correlate is the small intestine. All of the others except the Three-Heater have a specific organ associated with them. According to a translation by Dr. Porkert of an early Chinese text, the Three-Heater is the "commander-in-chief of the energies of all orbs . . . . If (the energy) of the *orbis tricalorii* is unimpeded, inside and outside, left and right, above and below are all in communication. Among (the functions) affecting the whole personality, pervading the body, harmonizing the interior and calming the exterior, developing on the left and sustaining on the right, conducting upward and communicating downward, none is more important than this." This essentially means that the network of our internal and external functioning is founded in, funded by, at the fundus of, the Three-Heater. The fluidity of communication and circulation in the kingdom is governed by this *san-chiao*. It is like the wise and true, amazingly enlightened and embracing old woman who makes sure everyone in the family has what they need to function at their very best. She encourages and empowers everyone in the family to their nature, to their purpose, giving each of them room to be themselves, to be at peace with their own nature, and to share their contribution to the natural movement of the Ch'i. In the *Ling-shu*, The Three-Heater is called an "orphaned" orb. (Porkert) It differs from the other orbs in regard to extension within the body. It has no form. It is more a context for life, than content. It is considered the medium of all communication—the fluidity of communication like waterways, open passages—communication among people, among the organ network of the body. The three *chiao* correspond to areas of the body, separate as three, connected as one—the upper *chiao*, middle *chiao* and lower *chiao*—but they do not correspond to particular organs except as the function of each organ is dependent upon the function of the Three-Heater.

As in all aspects of the life force, we can never define the Three-Heater once and for all, we can only share our experience and interpretations. The Three-Heater is a basic function. It is the keeper of Fire, therefore of light and warmth. It grants us the bearing of Fire, of light and warmth to others. It is the Bunsen burner for transformation as we dance in a broken world of division and deep union. The Three-Heater grants us to be alive, impassioned lovers of life as we engage with each other. Our entire chemistry requires heat to metabolize, to shift from one state to another, to complete its reactions. Fire grants our capacity to be warm and provide warmth. To be light and provide illumination is crucial to the fullness of our lives, crucial to the quality of every moment. All communication depends on our ability to share ourselves. This takes place best in an environment that is alive, perfect for life and open to the continuous movement that life is, an environment that we can enter into and where we can become one with all that is present.

The Three-Heater allows real meeting to take place. It is the promise-meeting in bodymindspirit, molecule to molecule, organ to organ, person to person, people to people. The meeting of I-Thou, a bonding between, with, among, us. "All real living is meeting." (Martin Buber) The very nature of relationship, of being related to one another is anchored in our origins. We reach for one another. There is an original and ongoing flow of life between us, I-Thou, Thou-I. What is required to further this flow is to recognize who we are. What separates us is our story. What unites us is that we are all interpreting, creating stories about ourselves and each other. Yet, we come to know who we are in each other's presence. We provide a healing presence for each other beyond the interpretations. We commune. This is the function in life associated with what the Chinese named *san-chiao*, Three-Heater. Further, this function speaks of the one who provides the milieu for wholeness, the great caretaker of life such that in the presence of each other's warmth and light we come to our own fullness of light and warmth. We come home, to the divine milieu, to the sacred fire, to the trinity of human being-heaven-earth, to the power that reconciles yes and no. We come home to that from which everything is born, in which everything is made one, toward which all life is directed.

There is a wonderful story to illustrate the great function of the Three-Heater as spacemaker, peacemaker, homemaker, caretaker, for all the rest of life. The story is from a little book called *The Sermon on the Mount According to Vedanta* by Swami Prabhavananda:

> In one of our monasteries there were a number of young postulants, not yet trained, fresh from school. When they had been together a short time, their old tendencies began to assert themselves, and the boys formed cliques and quarreled. A senior swami of our order went to investigate. He questioned everybody and soon discovered the ring-leaders. Then he wrote to Swami Brahmananda, who was the head of our order, that these boys were unfitted for monastic life and should be expelled. My master answered: "Don't do anything about it. I am coming myself." When he arrived at the monastery, he did not question anyone. He just started living there. He insisted on only one thing—that all the boys should meditate in his presence regularly every day. The boys soon forgot their quarrels. The whole atmosphere of the place became uplifted. By the time Swami Brahmananda left, two to three months later, perfect harmony had been established in the monastery. No one had to be expelled. The minds and hearts of the postulants were transformed.

The Three-Heater is the link, the hyphen between the universe and the human, between human and human, the firing of the vessel of self in the world, the place of meeting that living is. The Three-Heater provides the light necessary for transformation, provides the warmth for keeping the entire family together, for communication. It is the member of the family whose purpose is to give her life away. (Dr. Worsley personalized each of the functions as Officials in accordance with old Chinese charts showing little old sages performing different functions.) She is also the one who provides a life imperative to the others, a certain compelling insistence to give life our attention now, to not wait to become masterful, but in fact to be masterful in whatever task is at hand, simply by giving ourselves away. Let us not wait. Besides, what would we be waiting for? Perhaps, it does not take time to be home.

It is not for nothing that the Three-Heater is associated with the great movement of the *Wu Hsing* known as Fire. Fire is interpreted as the aspect of nature the source of which is the sun. What we say about nature we say about ourselves. We are the Sun, daystar, luminary, source of fire for life with each other. Our nature is to be alive, present to life, passionate, radiant, brilliant, joyfilled. We see and we touch by way of the sun's fire. Without illumination we can not see, without warmth we can not touch, without joy we can not trust in bodymindspirit. Fire is a life principle, a phenomenon to be reckoned with. It does not go unnoticed. It is urgent, fascinating, coercive, powerful, equalizing, necessary to sustain life. It compels us to attention immediately. It brings us to life directly. It gives itself away. It is dynamic. All of this am I, are you. We are interpretable as Fire. It is in this context that we speak of Three-Heater, the communicator of Fire, the minister of the sun. Without her we go cold, dark, joyless, dead. With her the whole kingdom is enlivened and in partnership. People laugh. Everyone is taken care of. Relationships flourish. The whole family functions with greatness, extraordinarily, *all twelve*: the Great Letting Go (X), the

Great Receiving (IX), the Great Transporting (XII), the Supreme Controller (I), the Great Heart Protector (V), the Great Master Architect (VIII), the Great Wise Decision Maker (Sophia) (VII), the Great Bringer to Fruition (XI), the Great Separator of Pure from Impure (II), the Great Conductor of the Vital Essence (IV), the Great Fluid Storehouse (III), and the Great Three-Heater (VI)—all come home. Each of them is a faculty of life, a specific power of acting, a conversation of the movement of human life. One might call them the twelve Great Conversations within which we live our life. These are conversations that govern life in our personal doing and our nonpersonal being.

At this moment we are exploring only one of these conversations—the Great Three-Heater. This is a wondrous promise of balance and harmony in the whole of the Kingdom, the teacher of the magnificence of human being.

> Go higher—Behold the Human Spirit
>
> — Sufi Poet

Given the nature of the Three-Heater, there is not one symptom of bodymindspirit that is not approachable or can not be touched through this pathway. Of the twenty-three points on the pathway, there are four points that are translated with the word "gate" as part of their name: VI 1, Rushing the Frontier Gate; VI 2, Fluid Secretion Gate; VI 5, Outer Frontier Gate; VI 21, Ear Gate. The Three-Heater is the keeper of the gates, the passageways. Pere Larre often interprets the gate as a gate in a field: when you consider it, there's no reason to have a gate in a wide open field except, perhaps, for the one making the passage—the gate reveals that one can make entrance. Gates are openings. Life requires openings. It could be said that life is an opening. All symptoms are a request to open. All symptoms are gates to pass through. Most of the pathways have at least one point that is a gate.

A path and a gateway have no meaning or use once the objective is in sight.

— A Sufi Teaching

Inside the Great Mystery that is,
we don't really own anything.
What is this competition we feel then,
before we go, one at a time, through the same gate?

— Sufi Poet

Some other categories of points along the pathways besides gates are ponds, streams, windows, palaces, paths, valleys, sources, halls, crossings, ducts, pivots, currents, springs, welcomes, ditches, borders, mountains, marshes, storehouses, mounds, pillars, bones, correspondences, meetings. All points are promises, invitations and requests. They give us access to ourselves. They "home" us.

I conclude this exploration of the Three-Heater for now, knowing it is infinitely interpretable. I give you two final readings, two interpretations, which speak to me of the nature of who we are as Fire, as _san-chiao_:

This is the true joy in life, the being used for a purpose recognized by yourself as a mighty one; . . . . the being a force of Nature instead of a feverish selfish little clod of ailments and grievances complaining that the world will not devote itself to making you happy . . . .

I am of the opinion that my life belongs to the community, and as long as I live, it is my privilege to do for it whatever I can. I want to be thoroughly used up when I die, for the harder I work the more I live. I rejoice in life for its own sake. Life is no "brief candle" to me. It is a sort of splendid torch which I have got hold of for a moment, and I want to make it burn as brightly as possible before handing it on to future generations . . . .

— Bernard Shaw

the lesson of the moth

i was talking to a moth
the other evening
he was trying to break into
an electric light bulb
and fry himself on the wires

why do you fellows
pull this stunt i asked him
because it is the conventional
thing for moths or why
if that had been an uncovered
candle instead of an electric
light bulb you would
now be a small unsightly cinder
have you no sense

plenty of it he answered
but at times we get tired
of using it
we get bored with the routine
and crave beauty
and excitement
fire is beautiful
and we know that if we get
too close it will kill us
but what does that matter
it is better to be happy
for a moment
and be burned up with beauty
than to live a long time
and be bored all the while
so we wad all our life up
into one little roll
and then we shoot the roll

that is what life is for
it is better to be a part of beauty
for one instant and then cease to
exist than to exist forever
and never be a part of beauty
our attitude toward life
is come easy go easy
we are like human beings
used to be before they became
too civilized to enjoy themselves

and before i could argue him
out of his philosophy
he went and immolated himself
on a patent cigar lighter
i do not agree with him
myself i would rather have
half the happiness and twice
the longevity

but at the same time i wish
there was something i wanted
as badly as he wanted to fry himself

— don marquis

References

Aiken, Robert. "The Body of the Buddha." Parabola, X, No. 3, August 1985.

Allen, Dick. *Overnight in the Guest House of the Mystic*. Baton Rouge: Louisiana State University Press, 1984.

Bergson, Henri. *The Two Sources of Morality and Religion*. Trans. R. Ashley Audra. Notre Dame, IN: University of Notre Dame Press, 1977.

Buckley, Thomas. "Living in the Distance." Parabola, IX, No. 3, August 1984.

Connelly, Dianne M. *Traditional Acupuncture: The Law of the Five Elements*. Columbia, MD: Centre for Traditional Acupuncture, 1974.

Cooper, J. C. *Yin and Yang*. Wellingborough, Great Britain: Aquarian Press, 1981.

Cummings, E. E. *Complete Poems*. New York: Harcourt Brace Jovanovich, 1972.

Da Free John. *Easy Death*. Clearlake, CA: The Dawn Horse Press, 1983.

De Mello, Anthony. *The Song of the Bird*. Garden City, NY: Image
Books, 1984.

Eliot, T. S. *Collected Poems, 1909-1962*. New York: Harcourt
Brace Jovanovich, 1970.

Frost, Robert. *The Poetry of Robert Frost*. Ed. Edward Connery
Lathem. New York: Holt, Rinehart and Winston, 1969.

Gilligan, Carol. *In A Different Voice*. Cambridge, MA: Harvard
University Press, 1982.

Ginsberg, Allen. *Collected Poems 1947-1980*. New York: Harper
and Row, 1984.

Hammarskjöld, Dag. *Markings*. Trans. Lief Sjoberg and W. H.
Auden. New York: Alfred A. Knopf, 1964.

Heidegger, Martin. *On the Way to Language*. New York: Harper
and Row, 1971.

Hoff, Benjamin. *The Tao of Pooh*. New York: E. P. Dutton, 1982.

Kazantzakis, Nikos. *Zorba the Greek*. New York: Simon and
Schuster, 1952.

Keller, Helen. *The Story of My Life*. Garden City, NY: Doubleday,
1902.

Kierkegaard, Søren. *Fear and Trembling* and *The Sickness Unto
Death*. Garden City, NY: Doubleday, 1954.

_____ . *Either/Or*. Garden City, NY: Doubleday, 1959.

Kinnell, Galway. *Mortal Acts, Mortal Words*. New York: Houghton
Mifflin, 1980.

Larre, Claude, and Elisabeth de la Vallée. *The Secret Treatise of
the Spiritual Orchid*. East Grinstead, Great Britain: British
Register of Oriental Medicine, 1985.

Larre, Claude, Jean Schatz, and Elisabeth de la Vallée. *Survey of Traditional Chinese Medicine*. Trans. Sarah Elizabeth Stang. Columbia, MD: Traditional Acupuncture Foundation, 1986.

Lao Tzu (Lao Tze). *Tao Teh Ching*. Trans. John C. H. Wu; ed. Paul K. T. Sih. New York: St. John's University Press, 1961.

Lawrence, D. H. *D. H. Lawrence: Selected Poems*. New York: Penguin Press, 1980.

Levine, Stephen. *Who Dies?* Garden City, NY: Anchor Books, 1982.

Lonergan, J. F. Bernard. *Insight: A Study of Human Understanding*. New York: Philosophical Library, 1957.

Lusseyran, Jacques. "Sense and Presence." *Parabola*, X, No. 3, August 1985.

Marquis, Don. *archy and mehitabel*. New York: Doubleday, 1927.

Maslow, Abraham. *Toward a Psychology of Being*. Princeton, NJ: Van Nostrand, 1968.

Maxwell, Florida-Scott. *The Measure of My Days*. New York: Alfred A. Knopf, 1979.

May, Rollo. *Freedom and Destiny*. New York: W. W. Norton, 1981.

Miller, Arthur. *After the Fall*. New York: Viking Press, 1964.

Milne, A. A. *The House At Pooh Corner*. New York: E. P. Dutton, 1928.

Naess, Arne. *Four Modern Philosophers*. Chicago: University of Chicago Press, 1968.

Ortega y Gasset, Jose. *What is Philosophy?* Trans. Mildred Adams. New York: Norton, 1960.

Paz, Octavio. *Configurations*. New York: New Directions, 1971.

Porkert, Manfred. *The Theoretical Foundations of Chinese Medicine*. Cambridge: The MIT Press, 1974.

Prabhavananda, Swami. *The Sermon on the Mount According to Vedanta*. Hollywood: Vedanta Press, 1963.

Reymond, Lizelle. "Intimate Journeys." *Parabola*, IX, No. 3, August, 1984.

Rilke, Rainer Maria. *The Selected Poetry of Rainer Maria Rilke*. Ed. and trans. Stephen Mitchell. New York: Random House, 1980.

Roethke, Theodore. *Straw for the Fire*. Ed. David Wagoner. Seattle, WA: University of Washington Press, 1980.

Schweitzer, Albert. *Out of My Life and Work*. London: Holt Allen, 1933.

Selzer, Richard. *Mortal Lessons: Notes on the Art of Surgery*. New York: Simon and Schuster, 1974.

Shaw, Bernard. "Epistle Dedicatory," *Man and Superman*. Copyright 1903 by Bernard Shaw. *Complete Plays*. New York: Dodd, Mead, 1963.

_____ . "Art and Public Money." Lecture at Brighton School of Art. Published in *Sussex Daily News* [Sussex, England], 7 March 1907.

Shaw, Indries. *The Way of the Sufi*. New York: E. P. Dutton, 1969.

Steiner, George. *Martin Heidegger*. New York: Penquin Press, 1978.

Stevens, Wallace. *The Collected Poems of Wallace Stevens*. New York: Alfred A. Knopf, 1967.

Tagore, Rabindranath. *Gitanjali*. Ed. Edmund R. Brown. Boston: International Pocket Library.

Teilhard de Chardin, Pierre. *Hymn of the Universe*. Trans. Simon Bartholomew. New York: Harper & Row, 1965.

Walker, Alice. *The Color Purple*. New York: Washington Square Press, 1982.

Watts, Alan. *Tao, The Watercourse Way*. New York: Pantheon Books, 1975.

————. *The Wisdom of Insecurity*. New York: Vintage Books, 1951.

Whitman, Walt. *Leaves of Grass*. New York: Doubleday, 1926.

Williams, Margery. *The Velveteen Rabbit*. New York: Holt, Rinehart and Winston, 1983.

Yeats, W. B. *The Collected Poems of W. B. Yeats*. New York: Macmillan, 1956.

Yourcenar, Marguerite. *Memoirs of Hadrian*. New York: Farrar, Straus and Giroux, 1954.